OXFORD MEDICAL PUBLICATIONS

Teaching Medicine in the Community

OXFORD GENERAL PRACTICE SERIES

Editorial Board

Godfrey Fowler, John Hasler, Jacky Hayden, Iona Heath, and Clare Wilkinson

Teaching Medicine in the Community

A Guide for Undergraduate Education

Oxford General Practice Series • 38

Edited by

CARL WHITEHOUSE

MARTIN ROLAND

and

PETER CAMPION

Universities of Manchester and Hull

OXFORD   TORONTO   MELBOURNE

OXFORD UNIVERSITY PRESS

1997

Oxford University Press, Great Clarendon Street, Oxford OX2 6DP

Oxford   New York

Athens   Auckland   Bangkok   Bogota   Bombay   Buenos Aires
Calcutta   Cape Town   Dar es Salaam   Delhi   Florence   Hong Kong
Istanbul   Karachi   Kuala Lumpur   Madras   Madrid   Melbourne
Mexico City   Nairobi   Paris   Singapore   Taipei   Tokyo   Toronto
and associated companies in
Berlin   Ibadan

Oxford is a trade mark of Oxford University Press

Published in the United States
by Oxford University Press Inc., New York

A catalogue record for this book is available from the British Library

Library of Congress Cataloging in Publication Data
Whitehouse, Carl.
Teaching medicine in the community: a guide for undergraduate
education / Carl Whitehouse, Martin Roland, and Peter Campion.
(Oxford general practice series; 38)
Includes bibliographical references and index.
1. Primary care (Medicine) – Study and teaching. 2. Community
health services – Study and teaching. 3. Primary care (Medicine) –
Study and teaching – Great Britain. 4. Community health services –
Study and teaching – Great Britain. I. Roland, M. O. (Martin
Oliver) II. Campion, Peter. III. Title. IV. Series.
R737.W74 1997   610'.71'1–dc20   96–30191   CIP

ISBN 0 19 262 653 1

Typeset by Palimpsest Book Production Limited,
Polmont, Stirlingshire

Printed and bound in Great Britain by
Biddles Ltd, Guildford and King's Lynn

Preface

Medical students have traditionally been taught clinical medicine by specialists in teaching hospitals. General practitioners recognized that their generalist role had a particular contribution to make and this has been reflected over the last forty years during student attachments to general practice. It is now recognized that the knowledge, skills, and attitudes gained by working with generalists in community settings have an importance for medical education which extends well beyond the discipline of general practice. This is reflected in the General Medical Council's most recent guidance on medical education. In addition to this, changes in medical practice, including shorter hospital stays and a stronger community base for many disciplines, are making it increasingly difficult to deliver traditional medical education within hospital settings.

For these two reasons, many medical schools are altering the balance of their courses to reflect a greater contribution from community-based disciplines. At the same time, medical schools are seeking to change their teaching methods, better to reflect the principles of adult learning. Students of the future will experience much less rote learning. A more critical approach to their own learning will prepare them better for a lifetime of learning. In many medical schools, academic general practitioners are at the forefront of these changes in educational method and content.

This book is for those involved as tutors in these new and developing courses. The book outlines the aims of community-based undergraduate teaching, describes in detail educational approaches that can be used, and summarizes methods for evaluation. Many tutors will come from general practice. The book describes the new types of experience that the student may expect to gain from attachments to the primary care team, with a much reduced emphasis on 'sitting and watching'. It recognizes the wide range of disciplines and resources within the community that will, in future, contribute to undergraduate education. However, we hope that the book will also be of value to hospital-based tutors, both in demonstrating how community-based attachments may be integrated with teaching within the hospital and in describing the principles and practice of new approaches to education, for example, small-group learning.

We hope that the book will provide, for new and old teachers alike, a balance between the theoretical and conceptual underpinning of the current changes in medical education and a practical guide to their implementation.

Many people have contributed, directly and indirectly, to the thinking of this book but we would particularly like to thank those who have contributed their innovative ideas in Part IV, and Lesley Southgate and Gareth Holsgrove for their fresh approach to assessment and evaluation in Part V.

Manchester   C.W.
September 1996   M.R.
                                                                                                        P.C.

Contents

List of contributors

David Adshead, Division of General Practice and Public Health Medicine, University of Leeds

Len Biran, Academic Unit of General Practice, University of Leeds

Dominic Blackie, Department of Primary Care, University of Liverpool

Paul Booton, Department of General Practice and Primary Care, King's College School of Medicine and Dentistry, London

Colin Bradley, Department of General Practice, The University of Birmingham

Peter Campion, Professor of Primary Care Medicine, Postgraduate Medical School, University of Hull

Joanna Collerton, Department of General Practice and Primary Care, King's College School of Medicine and Dentistry, London

Chris Dowrick, Department of Primary Care, University of Liverpool

Paramjit Gill, Centre for Research in Primary Care, University of Leeds

Susanna Graham-Jones, Department of Public Health and Primary Care, University of Oxford

Gareth Holsgrove, Associate Professor of Medical Education, United Arab Emirates University, Al-Ain, UAE

Diana Kelly, St Bartholomew's and the Royal London School of Medicine and Dentistry, London

Martin Lawrence, Department of Public Health and Primary Care, University of Oxford

Kieran McGlade, Department of General Practice, Queen's University Belfast

Nigel Oswald, Unit of General Practice, University of Cambridge

Martin Roland, Professor of General Practice, University of Manchester

Lesley Southgate, Professor of Primary Care and Medical Education, CHIME, The Whittington Hospital, University College Medical School, London

Carl Whitehouse, Professor of Teaching Medicine in the Community, University of Manchester

Geoff Wykurz, St Bartholomew's and the Royal London School of Medicine and Dentistry, London

Part One
Background

1 Introduction

Our modern doctrine is a contrivance of the word-catchers; the art of talking rather than the art of healing!

(Thomas Sydenham, *The works*, Vol. I)

Profound changes are taking place in health care provision throughout the world. These derive from factors as diverse as technological developments, the changing demography, and increasing involvement of consumers. The speed and extent of these changes have inevitably produced considerable stresses at the interface between education and provision. Many questions have arisen. Does medical education provide the kinds of professionals society will need in the 21st century? Do modern health care institutions provide suitable facilities to train the health workers of the 21st century?

One result of considering these questions has been a new revolution in medical education as significant as that introduced by Thomas Sydenham in the 17th century. Sydenham, known as the English Hippocrates, taught that observation should have precedent over theory in the management of disease. He was concerned that all his medical methods should be based on evidence. He encouraged training of the students' sight, hearing, and touch and experimental skills. He wanted to move beyond words to experience.

The new medical education emphasizes that the psychosocial context is as important as the biological processes in the understanding of illness. It is concerned that medicine should be based on a holistic approach. It encourages training students to listen to their patients, to be prepared to inform and negotiate.

In the last decade of the 20th century there has been a groundswell of structural and attitudinal change that has made it possible to implement new approaches. This has included a new focus on the role of the community in medical education, although the idea of community-based medical education itself is not new.

General practice is a key element in these community approaches in countries like the United Kingdom that have a strong tradition of practice-based primary care. General practice as a discipline has long been concerned with issues such as the psychosocial context of patients, consultation skills, and decision-making. The unique advantage of being responsible for defined populations has led general practices to be increasingly involved in aspects of population medicine such as epidemiology, needs assessment and health care organization. All these aspects make general practice a valuable resource for learning. At the same time there are many other demands on all community resources, and especially individual practices, which may make it difficult to grasp these opportunities.

The aim of this book is to help current and prospective teachers discover the needs, the opportunities, and the methods for education in the community. This will enable them to play a more effective role in facilitating the learning of medical students.

BACKGROUND

A historical perspective can usefully illuminate current developments in medical education. This section provides a brief review of developments in past centuries. It then considers the major influences on developments at the beginning of the 20th century and looks at the foundations of some radical developments in the last few decades. This provides a background to the current proposals for reform of medical education in the United Kingdom and the place that the community and general practice might play in this.

Historical perspective

Medical education has been part of human activity since the earliest recorded civilisations. Ancient Chinese medicine dates back to 2900 BC, with written records from the 8th century AD. Formal licensing also existed from this time, and organized schools from the 10th century AD. However, it was the Greek tradition, originating in the 6th century BC, which has had the greatest influence on the development of Western medicine. Greek medical education centred on teaching groups or 'schools'. By far the most famous was that of Hippocrates (460–?377 BC) on the island of Cos. In Greece, medicine was an art learnt by apprenticeship in which 'the neophyte received instruction, participated in the care of patients, assisted and nursed as needed, and performed menial tasks in maintaining the equipment as required by the teacher' (Lyons and Petrucelli 1987, p.196) and Hippocrates took students for training for which he charged a fee. What the Hippocratic tradition contributed above all was the clinical method in which history and physical examination were included. He wrote:

In order to prognosticate correctly who will recover and who will die, in whom the days will be long, in whom short, one must know all the symptoms, and must weight their relative value.

The patient's appearance is observed in detail . . . An ear is held to the chest to hear the breathing . . . palpation discloses the temperature as well as the characteristics of parts of the body.

(Lyons and Petrucelli 1987)

However, the psychosocial was not ignored:

No detail of a patient's appearance and function was to be omitted. Moreover his way of life, his emotional state, surroundings, and behaviour were carefully examined . . . the climate and customs of his city and country were also part of the medical examinations. (Lyons & Petrucelli 1987)

This tradition continued in many forms. An important development was in Arab medicine with its scholarly, clinical emphasis on describing and differentiating diseases seen. Throughout this long period medical practice was closely associated with teaching students to ensure the continuation of the profession.

The distinction between a 'medical school' and medical practice was more recent. The first European School of Medicine was founded at Salerno in Southern Italy, probably in the 9th century AD. It was highly influential in medieval Europe. It was at Salerno, in 1140, that Roger II of Sicily first insisted on examination and certification of physicians. In 1221, Emperor Frederick II went further and decreed that no one should practice medicine unless he had been examined by the masters of Salerno, after studying logic for three years, medicine and surgery for five, and after practising under the direction of an experienced physician for one further year! This pattern highlights the second strand in the development of medical education with its emphasis on theoretical knowledge. This strand was associated with the development of universities in many European cities from Padua to Oxford and Krakow from the 12th century AD. Here the study of classical writers such as Aristotle and physicians such as Galen and Avicenna, led to the development of systematic approaches to the theory of medicine. The writings from these three traditions (Greek, Roman, and Arab) were elevated to dogma and became the basis of university teaching. Many universities, including even Oxford and Cambridge, excluded any direct transmission of experience from practising physicians. Clinical teaching as part of a university medical course was uncommon until it was developed at Leiden in the early 18th century, followed by changes at the universities of Vienna and Edinburgh. Although the universities inhibited observational science, they did stress the importance of discipline and logic in approaching medical problems. Other branches of what was to become the medical profession (such as guilds of surgeons and apothecaries) continued to teach by apprenticeship. This led to considerable conflict between the branches.

The third strand in the development can be traced to the input of religious organizations (and in particular Christian communities) into providing hospitals and various orders to care for sick people, often away from their homes and communities. These concentrations of sick people provided a basis for the development of teaching hospitals. At the beginning of the 18th century, practical medical education in England was a matter of individual apprenticeships or was in the hands of individual doctors who ran their own private schools dealing with anatomy and surgery through lectures and demonstrations of dissection. The next move came with the founding of new hospitals to meet the growing demand of the poor for medical care. Many of the religious institutions had disappeared after the reformation although some, such as St Bartholomew's and St Thomas's, had been refounded. In the 18th century new hospitals were established: from Westminster Hospital in 1720 to the Radcliffe Infirmary at Oxford in 1770. It was natural for clinical teachers to congregate where there were groups of sick people and so many leading teachers became visiting physicians and surgeons to these new hospitals. Students began to receive clinical instruction by walking the wards observing their work. At first, the hospitals were concerned that time spent on education would detract from time spent on clinical work, but after a while it became clear that encouraging students was a good way to attract people to work in the hospitals. In 1785, William Blizard and James Maddock at the London Hospital obtained permission to build a medical school adjoining the hospital where students could receive lectures on the principles and theory of practice which would enable them to develop practical skills effectively. Thus, the first complete English medical school was founded (Ellis 1986). Other great medical schools (St Bartholomew's, St. Thomas's, Guys, St. George's, and the Middlesex) soon followed.

However, the universities still tended to draw some teachers of medicine away from treating the sick to places where they could study and theorize. In due course, hospitals were linked as teaching institutions with universities but even then a distinction was usually maintained between the basic scientific training (in disciplines such as anatomy and physiology) and the practical clinical training: the long-standing division between preclinical and clinical courses. This was particularly noticeable on the continent of Europe.

William Osler and Abraham Flexner

At the end of the 19th century, the physician William Osler (later to become Regius Professor of Medicine at Oxford) and the pathologist William Welch pioneered a new model of medical education at John Hopkins University School of Medicine, Baltimore. This so-called scientific model emphasized the need for a theoretical scientific basis to all disciplines, including the clinical disciplines, and led to a more rigorous approach to assessing clinical procedures and treatments. These reforms were slow to spread and in the early years of this century the American medical education reformer, Abraham Flexner, was commissioned by the Carnegie Foundation for the Advancement of Teaching to explore the quality of medical education in the United States. He first toured the medical school of the United Kingdom and Europe where he was impressed by many aspects of the organization and teaching that he saw in different situations (Flexner 1912). On the one hand, he commended the apprenticeship style of British clinical education at that time with the actual and continuous participation of the student in the care of the sick. He considered that 'in all that pertains to the relation of the student to the hospital, the English model deserves to be universally copied'. At the same time he was highly critical of the lack of a proper scientific base and he valued the combination of teaching and research in Germany with its strong scientific orientation. His later report on the situation in the United States and Canada led to the general adoption of the scientific model. At the same time it perpetuated the division between preclinical and clinical stages.

Osler himself, although a strong proponent of scientific approaches, had always been aware of the need for wider considerations as a quotation from his valedictory address at McGill University, where he moved after John Hopkins, shows:

Divide your attentions equally between books and men. The strength of the student of books is to sit still eating the heart of a subject with pencil and note-book in hand . . . The strength of a student of men is to travel—to study men, their habits, character, mode of life, their behaviour under varied conditions, their vices, virtues and peculiarities. (see Osler 1951)

At the time of the reforms in the United States, which also had a strong influence in other Western countries, Flexner's reasons were cogent. There is no doubt that the reforms were effective: his approach has had a resilience that has enabled it to last basically unchanged for 80 years.

The development of new approaches

In the last quarter century departures from this model have appeared. Many of these innovations have been associated with the emergence of new medical schools such as the University of Limburg, Maastricht; McMaster University, Hamilton, Ontario; and the University of Newcastle, New South Wales.

The founding of the medical school at Newcastle has been well described (Hamilton 1992; Reid 1993). It is a good example of the reasons behind a move onwards from the Flexnerian approach. It was a specific response to a government committee of enquiry into Medical Education and Manpower Needs in Australia which considered there were serious defects in the traditional methods of medical education. Graduates of the established medical schools were thought to be oriented too much towards the diagnosis and management of disease in individuals and not sufficiently sensitized to the psychosocial and community aspects of illness. Newcastle responded to the committee's concerns by developing a community-oriented curriculum with students given the opportunity to move outside hospital, to develop skills in approaching the community, and to talk to people within it. General practice had a major role within the community disciplines and the whole curriculum but it was stressed that the intention was 'to produce doctors who could enter all varieties of medical practice with a broad understanding of medicine and of community health'.

Some Third World settings with concerns for large and poorly served rural populations have also been innovative in considering how the teaching and practice of medicine should be adapted in different communities (King 1966; Monekosso 1993). Recently, this work has been encouraged through the Network of Community-oriented Educational Institutions for Health Sciences, based in Maastricht, which aims to promote innovation of education in the health professions and address it to the health needs of societies.

Although the founding of new schools in the United Kingdom, at Nottingham and Southampton, led to some innovations, there has been difficulty in developing these. It is even more recently that experimental courses have been tried within long-established schools such as Cambridge, London, Liverpool, and Manchester.

This brief historical overview suggests that there are a number of key issues in developing good medical education:

- response to the needs and expectations of the society served;
- balancing a knowledge of diseases with an understanding of the reallife situation of patients;
- balancing theoretical input with practical experience;
- accepting the need to critically observe and experiment so that practical experience is scientifically based;
- ensuring that students, teachers, and patients can be brought together in a suitable environment.

Many of these issues have re-emerged in the current educational developments. Some of the impetus for these has come from the radical changes in the nature of health care since 1990.

CHANGES IN MEDICAL EDUCATION IN THE UNITED KINGDOM

The GMC and its recommendations

For nearly 150 years, the General Medical Council of the United Kingdom (GMC) has been responsible for ensuring that doctors are properly qualified. One part of this obligation has been to monitor the education and the examination of doctors. Every 10 years the GMC has produced recommendations on undergraduate medical education.

In 1993, after a prolonged period of discussion, a series of radical recommendations was produced in the document *Tomorrow's doctors* (GMC 1993). In this document, which is further discussed in Chapter 3, the GMC was not just building on previous reports, nor simply responding to the many changes in health care provision in Britain. It was responding to major educational pressures which are being felt throughout the world.

There is no doubt that there is an international climate of change in medical education. Increased medical mobility, for instance within the European Union, is bringing different educational cultures in contact with each other and British medical education is not isolated from this. Many of these issues were discussed at a World Summit on Medical Education in 1993 (Walton 1993). There have been different responses. The Dutch, for instance, have developed an extensive national *Blueprint* (Metz *et al.* 1994), which details what is to be expected of a doctor who completes undergraduate education. The profile of the medical graduate is very similar to that produced in *Tomorrow's doctors*, but in *Blueprint* it is used to develop much more complex objectives ranging from global knowledge of the financial aspects of health care to the ability to cope with uncertainty and from the recognition of abnormalities and symptoms to recording in a testable, unambiguous, and readable manner. The Dutch authors also listed about 400 problems as starting points for training that ranged from alopecia to abnormality of the foot, and from poor weight gain in pregnancy to problems with loneliness.

The British approach has been less directive although it included the need to review both the curriculum and the methods of teaching. The authors of *Tomorrow's doctors* looked at many areas, but they were particularly concerned about:

- the continued overcrowding of the curriculum and excessive information load;
- the need to develop attitudes to learning based on enquiry and the exploration of knowledge.

They felt that the best way of dealing with these problems was to reduce radically the amount of information students were required to learn but at the same time 'strive to educate doctors capable of adaptation to change, with minds that can encompass new ideas and developments and with attitudes to learning that inspire the continuation of the educational process throughout professional life'.

A major emphasis of the GMC recommendations was a review of what the newly qualified doctor should be expected to be able to do as they enter the pre-registration year. The old idea that a doctor at qualification 'possessed the knowledge and skill requisite for the efficient practice of medicine, surgery, and midwifery' was laid to rest after a hundred years. It was now accepted that the undergraduate years do not lead to an end-point, but only to a node on a continuum of learning that passes on through general professional training, vocational specialist training, higher professional training, and the continuing education of a lifetime. This concept of the student as a lifelong learner implied a new view of the educational process. Consideration of how to maintain educational curiosity from undergraduate days throughout professional life was required.

Changes in educational approach

The concept of the undergraduate as an active learner is being rediscovered throughout the University system. For some time an emphasis developed on collecting facts and regurgitating them at set-points called examinations. In this system there is a danger that the facts are never absorbed and integrated into the student's experience. As many such facts are apparently never required again after the examination there is a considerable danger of what is termed passive, surface learning. Higher Education teachers are now seeking to develop a more active approach to learning. In this approach there are four distinctive features (Denicolo *et al.* 1992):

1. Students are involved in searching for personal and academic meaning to their studies in order to gain a sound grasp of key concepts and are able to analyse, reflect, and apply them.
2. Students are given greater responsibility for their own learning, being challenged to think things through for themselves, to identify and tackle problems, and to discuss ideas with others.
3. A high priority is put on acquiring skills and not just a body of knowledge. In particular, this applies to skills in problem-solving, interaction, and communication.
4. Students are encouraged to look beyond the immediate programme of study towards the challenges of their subsequent careers and everyday lives.

Application of these four principles has been particularly important in medical education. First, it has led to the development of integrated courses, as described in Chapter 2, where students are not taught in tightly knit blocks of anatomy, pathology, or surgery. Instead, they start from a problem or a case and are encouraged to explore what they need to learn in order to understand and manage that problem. They realize they need to explore basic, pathological, and clinical sciences if they are going to achieve this understanding. In this way, they absorb appropriate facts and develop an understanding for the relevance of many of the basic principles of these sciences to their future career. At the same time, they are involved in a process that develops their skills in problem-solving. This process also helps them to acquire other skills and attitudes, such as library skills or a critical approach to received wisdom.

Second, there is an emphasis on group learning. Lecture-based courses are not only more passive but they emphasize individual learning. Responsibility for one's own learning does not mean that one has to be the isolated book-student that Osler described. The new approaches emphasize the value of the team or group. Groups provide the opportunity for sharing, testing, and deepening knowledge. At the same time, students can learn interactional and communication skills.

Third, application of these principles means a greater emphasis on skills development. In medical education this has led to the development of 'skills laboratories' alongside the traditional institutions of hospital, medical school, and community, as described in Chapter 8. Within skills laboratories a range of new resources may be available including anatomical models for training in manual and examination skills, standardized patients for developing skills in professional communication, and interactive information technology for developing problem-solving and understanding.

Fourth, and most importantly, students are encouraged to develop study skills that can be used throughout their career because they have to carry out vocational training and keep up to date in the midst of a hectic professional life and because they have to cope with the rapidly changing theatre of medicine.

General practice has long been in the forefront of educational thinking in medicine. It was the first discipline with a defined structure for vocational training. This was backed up by considerable thought about educational content and method in both the development of vocational training courses and in individual trainer—trainee relationships (RCGP 1970; Byrne and Long 1975). As general practitioners became increasingly involved in undergraduate training they were able to bring these skills and knowledge with them.

GENERAL PRACTICE AS AN ACADEMIC DISCIPLINE

When the UK National Health Service (NHS) started in 1948 general practice had no place in medical education. During the first decade of the NHS a few key individuals realised that students needed to have experience outside the hospital walls and that this experience could be arranged through exposure to general practice.

Early developments and the foundation of the RCGP

These early developments are associated with Richard Scott's work in Edinburgh. As early as 1948, he set up a unit for teaching general practice which was not concerned with vocational training. In his own words 'it provided an opportunity for senior students to be confronted with a patient—doctor situation which the student could resolve only by integrating for himself a great deal of what he had learnt elsewhere'. (WMA 1954)

In 1954, Darbishire House Health Centre was set up in Manchester with the following aims:

• First-class medical care for the inhabitants of a densely populated city area.
• A demonstration of the proper integration of preventive and curative services as

represented by the personal health services of the local authority, the family practitioner services, and the hospital specialist services.

* An instrument for undergraduate medical education which can be used to leaven the present emphasis given to hospital medicine.
* The means of showing how medical care can take into account the social factors in the causation of disease in the individual and the community, thus demonstrating the use of such a centre as an instrument of socio-medical research.

A key development of this period was the foundation of The Royal College of General Practitioners in 1952. The College proposed at its foundation that there should be a department of general practice in each medical school in the United Kingdom. This view was supported by Sir Henry Cohen at the First World Conference on Medical Education in 1953:

But the synoptic view is not simply of man as an individual 'extracted from his realm' and treated as 'a thing apart'. It sees man also as a member of a family and as a unit in society. In the days when apprenticeship formed part of the medical student's training many social aspects of medicine could be culled from daily experiences in the patient's home. Today we must still provide for this experience in our undergraduate curriculum; not better to prepare the undergraduate for general practice, but to give him a balanced view of medicine as a single discipline. (Sir Henry Cohen, (WMA 1954))

The College was concerned about all educational matters although there was a particular emphasis on postgraduate training. A seminal book in the development of education in the field was *The future general practitioner* (RCGP 1972). This included a job definition for a general practitioner (Box 1) which, although since modified, contained ideas which could blossom as medical practice changed. Many of these concepts, such as making diagnoses in physical, psychological, and social terms, and working in a team, are now central to community-oriented education.

University departments of general practice

The early support of the (Royal) College of General Practitioners for university units in the discipline continued but was slow in being put into effect. Departments of

---

Box 1   The job definition of a general practitioner (from RGCP 1972, p.1)

The general practitioner is a doctor who provides personal, primary and continuing medical care to individuals and families. He [*sic*] may attend his patients in their homes, in his consulting-room or sometimes in hospital. He accepts the responsibility for making an initial decision on every problem his patient may present to him, consulting with specialists when he thinks it appropriate to do so. He will usually work in a group with other general practitioners, from premises that are built or modified for the purpose, with the help of paramedical colleagues, adequate secretarial staff and all the equipment which is necessary. Even if he is in single-handed practice he will work in a team and delegate when necessary. His diagnoses will be composed in physical, psychological and social terms. He will intervene educationally, preventively and therapeutically to promote his patient's health.

Community Medicine or Social Medicine (now Public Health) had long existed, but these departments could not provide clinical learning about individuals in a community. The first Department of General Practice was not established until 1957 (Edinburgh) and in 1968 this was still the only independent department. Four years later this had at last grown to six and the development had really begun (Byrne 1973).

In the 1960s, many medical school students were allowed to choose to spend a short elective period in general practice in their final clinical years. However, by 1968 less than half the medical schools arranged for all students to be taught in general practice. It was not always clear what the educational objectives of these attachments were and general practitioners (GP) teachers were not always paid even an honorarium. The main responsibility of the small departments of general practice was often to organize the attachments and possibly arrange some briefing and evaluation. However, as academic departments grew so they naturally developed their own research base. This base provided an understanding of their core concerns within an undergraduate course. The Association of University Departments of General Practice (AUDGP) was formed and continues to provide an important forum for developing research and education within the discipline.

Many of the full-time appointments to these Departments were people who had previously been in service practice and had developed educational expertise within the field of vocational training. Many other GPs were associated with Departments on a part-time basis and a large proportion of these also worked as trainers or course organizers. This provided a major resource of educational expertise.

By the mid 1990s there were Academic Units of General Practice in all British medical schools although some of these were still subunits of other departments. These units are increasingly concerned about education in primary health care, a holistic approach to patients and the influence of community and environment. They often take a major role in communication-skills teaching and are beginning to take a much greater part in teaching other basic clinical skills. Medical schools have become aware that they are a gateway to a major resource for educational expertise and facilities.

General practice is not, of course, the only discipline working within the community, although there is no doubt that the educational interest and expertise of general practice are of key importance in community-based education. Consideration of medical student education in the community must consider also the input from departments, such as psychiatry and paediatrics, and from other health professionals and other sectors. Of particular importance is the input from public health.

PUBLIC HEALTH AND GENERAL PRACTICE

Public health is another discipline which has changed considerably in recent years. Many of the developments have paralleled changes in general practice and many public health skills are now seen as important within general practice. These include epidemiology, needs assessment, and health promotion. General practitioners were already prepared to 'intervene educationally, preventively and therapeutically to promote a patient's health'. This conforms with the role of primary health care as perceived by the World Health Organization (WHO 1987) and follows an international trend. It is true that, in Britain, general practice-based primary health care is still largely 'medicine-centred' rather than 'health-centred' However, a new public health approach sees interventions with individuals and within communities through the structures of primary health care as a major contribution to the promotion of health (Ashton and Seymour 1988).

Primary care remains the educational field where medical students can best assess how their future professional role relates to other health inputs. It is here also that they can discover and evaluate the tension between the population-based approach of public health and the needs of individuals. Three areas briefly illustrate this.

1. Prevention

The spread of HIV infection in many countries over the last 15 years has been a reminder of how rapidly the health status of a society can be shaken. Curative approaches may have little part to play in control and the importance of preventive approaches is shown. Another example of the need to move beyond curative approaches is the 'epidemic' of heart disease. This has been particularly shown in former communist countries where there has even been a decrease in life expectancy, with increased cardiovascular deaths and concerns about smoking, alcohol consumption, and pollution. Doctors of the future need to be aware of the principles of disease prevention and health promotion even if the necessary approaches lie more in the field of education or environmental change. This will enable them to make a realistic contribution to discussions on resource allocation as well as to advising and helping individuals, families, and communities.

The idealistic view, expressed by the American physician, William Mayo, is that 'the aim of medicine is to prevent disease and prolong life, the ideal of medicine is to eliminate the need of a physician' (Mayo 1928). Other writers have questioned the value of many of the screening and health promotion activities carried out by doctors. It is important for future health professionals to be able to make a critical assessment of this (cf. Skrabanek and McCormick 1992). There is no doubt that it is on the political agenda in most countries. For instance, the British Government has said that it 'intends positively to encourage family doctors and primary health care teams to increase their contribution to the promotion of good health' (HMSO 1987).

2. Demographic change and disability

Increasing life expectancy has been associated with a change in the pattern of disease in the community. Old age is beset by disabilities resulting from chronic disease. Many of these disabilities might have been prevented earlier. Partial success in other areas of medical care (from prenatal care to resuscitation) has also provided some people who continue to bear chronic burdens of disability and disease. Many advances have been made in reversing disease processes and replacing body parts but people still suffer from considerable chronic disability that cannot be cured. Public health approaches to limit the handicap from such disabilities are as important as relief of symptoms or other medical interventions. These approaches include environmental and social change. Doctors for the 21st century need to learn about rehabilitation in this wider context.

3. Consumerism

A third area of change is the growth of what has been termed 'consumerism'. In the past, doctors, working under the ethical principle of beneficence, were expected to do the best for their patients. In a sense patients were 'expected' to accept that. A mystique surrounded the skill and the status of doctors. Patients lacked the knowledge to contest what doctors said. In many cases, doctors were seen as social superiors who should not be contradicted. A patient lying in bed in pain and distress will still want a powerful doctor to come and relieve their suffering: this is unsurprising and reasonable. However, in most other circumstances the position has rightly changed. Most doctor—patient contacts take place in ambulant situations (general practices or out-patients) where the patient is well enough in control, despite any anxiety or pain, to wish to be an equal partner in the discussion with the doctor. The development of Patient Charters is just one way of encapsulating the patient's right to be involved. Doctors now recognize and respond to the principle of personal autonomy.

Similar principles can be applied to assessing the health needs of a whole community, which public health physicians would call making a community diagnosis, and involving the community in that process. Here, there is a greater difficulty of defining the boundaries of a community and offsetting the needs of different groups within it. Concepts such as cost-effectiveness may need to be balanced against consumer demand. The principles of equity and personal autonomy can conflict.

CHANGES IN PROVISION OF HEALTH CARE IN THE UNITED KINGDOM

The General Medical Council noted how external factors relating to perceptions of health and health care would influence medical education. These factors are diverse ranging from the increased emphasis on prevention of disease and the new ethical issues surrounding the growth of consumerism, mentioned above, to the advent of new clinical and information technology and the redistribution of tasks between different health care professionals.

Reforms in the National Health Service

The early 1990s in the United Kingdom saw a complete revolution in the organization and provision of health care, initiated by three major documents from the government: *Promoting better health, Working for patients,* and *Caring for People* (HMSO 1987, 1989*a, b*). As their names suggest, two were on promoting better health through primary care and care in the community. The third (*Working for patients*) began the major financial restructuring in what became known as the purchaser—provider split. In many ways, this revolution was no more than a response to changes already occurring in the provision of care in many countries. Four areas are of particular relevance to the provision of medical education.

1. A primary care-led NHS

A key advancement in general practice in the United Kingdom has been the concept of a 'primary care-led NHS'. Whether through fund-holding or newer ideas of commissioning the so-called gatekeeper role of general practice has changed. This has meant that much more of early investigation and even treatment of patients is now kept 'outside the gate' of secondary care. Outside the gate is therefore the place where students have the opportunity to learn.

2. Care in the community

General practice has clearly always been concerned with providing 'continuing medical care to individuals and families'. As scientific medicine expanded, management of long-term illness became a prerogative of secondary care in hospitals. The development of chronic disease clinics with the use of practice nurses and protocols has once again altered this. The application in England and Wales, from 1993, of the Community Care aspects of the National Health Service and Community Care Act 1990 also brought changes. Increasingly, patients with long-term problems are maintained at home rather than in hospital. The development of nursing-home care in place of long-stay wards has altered the balance between general practice care and hospital care. A student who needs to learn about the natural history of disease and its effects on patients and their families will need to learn in the community.

3. The GP and the consumer

The move to consumerism discussed above could be seen as part of the concept of providing personal care and accepting the responsibility for what patients present. Doctors need to realize that the patient's wider needs and health beliefs are going to affect the interactions that take place and therefore they need to listen to patient views. This has been termed 'meetings between experts' (Tuckett *et al.* 1985) and emphasizes the need to explore and conceptualize the key elements in the patient's way of thinking.

General practice has long been concerned with this need to determine the patient's beliefs, concerns, and expectations, which was formulated by Pendleton and his colleagues (Pendleton *et al.* 1984) as one of the tasks of an ideal consultation. Such an approach showed that teaching communication was as much a matter of cultivating attitudes, such as the desire to be patient-oriented, as developing specific interpersonal skills. This has added a further aspect to the training that medical students should get in communication and history-taking. It has also moved much ethical learning away from major philosophical discussions on subjects such as abortion and euthanasia, and towards questions of the interrelationship between personal autonomy, beneficence and equity, and the problems that occur in negotiating what is right for an individual.

4. Technological change

Technological developments have completely altered the ways doctors can investigate and treat many patients. The 'Future general practitioner' (Royal College of General Practitioners 1972) spoke of the 'equipment which is necessary', but at the time this was quite basic. Irvine (1972) found that in many teaching practices it was limited to vaginal speculum, proctoscope, refrigerator, sterilizer, and minor surgery equipment. At that time, half had a microscope and one in three a haemoglobinometer, neither of which would be common today, showing the changes in approach to investigation. However, the development of electronic equipment and miniaturization have greatly increased the technical capabilities within general practice.

Changes in imaging methods and the introduction of new surgical techniques have enabled many more patients to be investigated and treated without having to be admitted to hospital even for one night. This will develop further over the next few years and many investigations may be devolved to centres outside hospitals, variously termed Primary Care Resource Centres or Diagnostic Centres, to which GPs have access. The coming of videotechnology and improved information technology links will mean that more diagnostic investigation and consultation can take place at a distance. These changes will also mean it is more difficult for students within an institution to meet and examine patients themselves.

BRINGING TOGETHER THE NEW APPROACHES IN HEALTH CARE AND EDUCATION

General practice has been at the forefront of the response to the changes in health care provision. It now provides new opportunities for undergraduate learning. However, the medical schools and hospitals still have their responsibilities and both settings are relevant. The major question is how best to deploy educational resources. There are two major pressures for a transfer of education into community settings. These may be termed the 'educational reasons' and the 'logistic reasons'.

Educational reasons

In view of the previous discussion it could be argued that the community is the appropriate setting for basic medical education. However, even totally community-based curricula (such as that described by Oswald in Part IV, Chapter 21) incorporate some access to hospitals, commonly linked to patients first encountered in the community. A full understanding of medicine cannot be obtained without experience within hospitals. It is necessary to consider what each site is best able to provide in terms of knowledge and experience.

The community provides access to a more 'normal' sector of society, to more common and more long-term health problems, to prevention and public health. Within the community it is much easier to obtain a holistic overview of patients and their health needs. Problems can be seen from the time they first present to the doctor until final resolution by recovery or death; problems can be seen within the psychosocial and environmental contexts; problems can be seen from the perspective of all the participants—health professionals and carers alike. Within the community it is also easier to look at the uncertainties surrounding medical care: the wide range of possibilities with the first presenting symptom, the wide range of problem-solving approaches, and the wide range of possible interventions and results.

However, within hospitals it is easier to look at the definitive signs and symptoms of disease entities and the practical aspects of interventions. It is also easier to focus on specific areas of knowledge and skills that might be required.

Logistic reasons

Educationally, it would appear that the resources available should be deployed in different settings in order for students to learn what is most appropriate in each situation. However, there are now a decreased number of hospital beds and patients spend a shorter time in hospital. These produce logistic pressures on hospital resources. Many aspects, which could be effectively taught in hospital, now need to be taught in the community because that is where the patients are. The patients are, of course, within the community at large and not waiting at health centres for students to learn, so there is always some preparation necessary if students are to receive focused education. For instance, if a student needs to learn the basic skills of heart auscultation they can certainly learn the normal hearts sounds on any (willing) patient who attends the surgery: they could just as easily learn these on each other. If their ability to pick up abnormal sounds is to be extended then they will need to see patients who have been brought in especially for the session.

The availability of tutors and resources in the community has also to be weighed. Community tutors need to assess whether to restrict their involvement to areas which can best or can only be taught in general practice, or whether they can and should become involved in helping to educate in areas which have traditionally been the remit of hospital departments.

If both community and hospital resources are to be used, there is the possibility of considerable overlap. There is, therefore, a role for shared teaching. In the past, much general practice involvement has been on a one-to-one basis with students in individual practices coupled with some seminar work within departments of general practice. An integrated approach which helps students develop a broader view of patients, and to develop better problem-solving skills may require the opportunity for the students to have access to the resources of primary care doctors and specialists at the same time. Many medical schools will be looking at the development of group-learning. This will be an area in which many community tutors will want to be involved in the future, even sharing the facilitation of a group with a hospital-based tutor.

Increased teaching requires financial resources. The days when it was considered a privilege to be sent a student and when doctors would provide teaching for little or no payment other than expenses have rightly disappeared. The corollary of that approach was that the teaching was an optional extra to be fitted in if there were no greater demands, otherwise the student would have to make do and learn as best they could. A major educational change has been the emphasis on evaluating the input and ensuring that students are enabled to achieve their goals. Educational developments must lead to improved skills, attitudes, and knowledge. Changes in the way that education is financed in the United Kingdom mean that in future all educational input will be monitored. Teaching that fails to meet appropriate standards will be discontinued. Once again, general practice has already experienced this in the selection and accreditation of training practices. In the United Kingdom, all teaching will in future be funded from two sources: either through the university funds and payments; or through the Service Increment for Teaching (SIFT) or its equivalents in other parts of the United Kingdom. Universities will have a major say in setting the contracts for SIFT allocation, and therefore in the monitoring. They will be expected to check not only that agreed services are provided but that educational objectives are met. Students themselves will be involved in this monitoring. They will want to know that they have learnt the art of healing rather than just a mass of words!

SUMMARY AND OVERVIEW OF OTHER PARTS OF THIS BOOK

Part I has looked at the historical background and the way that current changes in educational approach and in health care are influencing developments in medical education. Although the focus has been on changes in the United Kingdom, the same principles are at work throughout the world. We have shown the increased opportunities and challenges for undergraduate learning in the community and how general practice will play a major part in this.

Part II begins with a brief review of educational theory. This is followed by chapters that consider curriculum design and the important issue of setting educational aims and objectives for a course.

Part III turns to individual teaching methods. It looks at how the needs of individual students can be assessed and how this can be linked to setting personal objectives for them. It then considers methods of teaching in different situations: the consulting room, at home, attachments to other members of the primary health care team, in small groups, in the lecture theatre, and in the skills laboratory. The later chapters provide practical advice on how to tie in the individual approaches to the achievement of various objectives.

Part IV looks at innovations in community-based education. Eleven different authors describe their own recent innovations and how these are being evaluated. Many of them are still 'work in progress' and have not yet been fully evaluated. The intention of this section of the book is to inspire readers to develop their own ideas rather than to provide blueprints.

Part V describes approaches to assessment and evaluation with particular concern for those that are applicable within the community-based curriculum.

A full list of references is available at the end of the text.

Part Two

What is to be learned and when?—setting objectives

Education cannot be succesfully pursued unless there exists at least some notion of the end-product which is desired.

(James McCormick 1992)

The first stage of any educational activity is to consider what the students need to learn. Part II discusses the content of an undergraduate medical course from a community perspective. The general aims of a medical education and how the community can contribute to these are discussed against a background of basic educational theory and course design. This is followed by a consideration of how needs of individual students can be assessed and a focus given to particular educational experiences. Part II concludes with a chapter that outlines a range of specific objectives achievable in a community setting.

2 Contemporary approaches to education and learning

Education is the process of promoting a change in what people can do. The purpose of education (from the Latin *ex*, out of and *ducere*, to lead) is to *lead* the learner from one state to another: from ignorance to knowledge, from incompetence to competence, from indifference to enthusiasm. Changes in a learner's state of mind, whether it be their knowledge, emotions, or attitudes, can only be inferred from their behaviour which is their observable activity. The students' performance, whether in formal tests of knowledge, in practical examinations or in everyday activities, is used to judge what they have learnt.

GOALS, AIMS, AND OBJECTIVES

In order for this change to be purposeful and directed, the educator (who can, in the case of self-directed learning, also be the learner) must have a clear view of the desired destination. This may be termed an *aim*, a *goal*, or an *objective*. Aims and goals usually describe the broad purpose of an educational process. Sometimes such statements can appear almost meaningless (e.g. 'The aim of undergraduate medical education is to produce a basically competent doctor'), although even such statements help to set outer boundaries (i.e. 'The aim of undergraduate medical education is to produce a basically competent doctor—and not a biological scientist, surgeon, or general practitioner'). However, a more useful approach is to have clear statements of the behaviours and competencies that have to be gained in order to attain this aim. Hence the concept has arisen of *educational objectives* (see Box 1).

Educational activities can be various components of a course from a single tutorial or clinical encounter through medium-term components, such as a week or a block, to

---

Box 1 Educational objectives

An educational objective is an explicit statement of an achievement which a student will be expected to have reached by means of an educational activity

---

a whole module or even the full course. Objectives should be set for each of these. The definition also emphasizes achievements: these must be susceptible to testing. The success of education can only be judged fairly if assessments are closely related to and, ideally, derived from previously set objectives. Objectives should therefore be stated in concrete and unambiguous terms and should include an indication of *when* the objective is to be achieved, such as 'At the end of the session, (or block or year) students will . . .'.

An educational objective is therefore like a radio beacon. Radio beacons have dual functions as an aid to air navigation: they show the pilot the direction a plane should be pointed and they act as a position marker for each stage of a flight. Educational objectives have dual functions as an aid to learning; they show the learner the direction to go and they act as achievement markers for each stage of a course.

WHY SET SPECIFIC OBJECTIVES?

There are benefits for the student, for the teacher, and for the institution, in having clearly stated objectives for a course, and for each part.

Learners benefit by having boundaries set for their work. The sum of all knowledge in a discipline such as medicine is now so vast that students easily feel overwhelmed at the thought of having to master it. If their goals are set realistically, in the form of objectives, then they should be able to approach a course or module with some confidence that they will be able to succeed. Students can plan their self-directed study with a greater sense that they are on the right lines. This benefit extends to the assessment of students' performance since, having defined the objectives, the scope of the assessment is automatically also defined.

Objectives help tutors, particularly those who have not been involved in the design of a course (such as general practitioners teaching in their practices), to know what is and is not required. There is a strong temptation to concentrate on topics which happen to be of great interest to the tutor but are not part of the curriculum, to the exclusion of essential, but perhaps less exciting, matters. Clear and comprehensive objectives can help teachers avoid presenting extraneous information. This applies to whatever format is being used: lecture or clinical session; handout or reading list.

Finally, evaluation of courses is made far easier if explicit objectives are available. These can be compared with external norms (such as the GMC recommendations in the case of medicine). Their relevance, feasibility, and clarity can be judged. The teaching and learning methods can be set against each objective. This process is becoming standard as the HEFCE (Higher Education Funding Council for England) requires regular quality assessment of teaching in universities.

To understand the various types of objectives that may need to be set it is necessary to consider the domains of education.

THE DOMAINS OF EDUCATION

Bloom (1965) was the first to formally classify educational objectives into three domains. Each domain contains a hierarchy of learning, from the simplest to the most complex:

(1) cognitive (knowledge, interpretative and problem-solving skills);
(2) psychomotor (perceptual and manual skills);
(3) affective (feelings, emotions, attitudes, interpersonal, and communication skills).

These are usually abbreviated, somewhat imprecisely, as 'knowledge, skills, and attitudes'. However, as achievement in different domains may require different educational methods, it is often helpful to recall the original terms to avoid misclassifying a particular objective.

In the past, medical educators have emphasized the cognitive, and to a lesser extent the psychomotor, components of learning while rarely addressing the important third, affective, domain. *Tomorrow's doctors*, the latest report by the Education Committee of the General Medical Council (GMC 1993) seeks to alter this balance by emphasizing the relationship between attitudes and 'high standards of practice' (see below).

Awareness of these three domains can help us analyse educational activity. Consider these questions:

• What factors influence learning in each domain?
• In the knowledge domain how does a learner move from a state of ignorance to the ability to recall propositions, and from the ability to recall to an understanding of the relationship between objects and the ability to synthesize new propositions?
• How do the three domains interrelate: for example, how does knowledge of cardiac physiology affect learning the skill of cardiopulmonary resuscitation, or how does an approach to learning based on curiosity (an objective in the affective domain) affect learning about the organization of a health service?

LEARNER-CENTRED EDUCATION

The last question points towards a major concern of modern medical education. The GMC justified its recommendations for a major revision of British undergraduate medical curricula on the grounds that 'attitudes to learning that are based on enquiry and the exploration of knowledge are dulled by an excessive information load . . .' and 'The student should also acquire and cultivate the ability to work independently . . . [and] . . . must therefore have a certain amount of free time for private study and self education throughout the curriculum. (GMC 1993 p.5)

To achieve such 'self-education', and develop attitudes of curiosity and discovery, a different approach to learning is needed. Until recently, much medical education followed the pattern of an older pupil—teacher model that used to be found in schools, where teachers set the curriculum and 'taught' by lecture, demonstration, and directed exercises. This 'didactic', fact-based pattern of education (sometimes called 'paedagogy') has been substantially replaced, even in schools, by more flexible approaches. Pupils are now often encouraged to 'find out' for themselves, using a range of resources. They are also encouraged to solve problems rather than simply acquire facts. Many students will have experienced this newer, liberal approach, called 'heuristic', or 'discovery learning'. A model drawing on this 'discovery learning', and also on the theoretical work of Carl Rogers and Donald Schön, is more useful for young adults who aspire to be self-regulating professionals. This approach is sometimes called 'androgogy' but is better described as 'learner-centred education' (Coles 1994).

LEARNING STYLES AND APPROACHES

Studies of how students approach learning show that different methods are adopted. These can be summarized as 'surface', 'deep', and 'strategic' processing (Newble and Entwistle 1986):

- *Surface processing* is associated with mere recall of facts. It is a memorizing or rote-learning approach.
- *Deep processing* occurs when students attempt to understand the meaning of what they are learning. It is associated with the synthesis of the information into meaningful material which is then related to a relevant context.
- *Strategic processing* is a hybrid of these; it is more calculating, directly related to immediate needs such as passing an examination.

Underlying motivations will affect these different behaviours. Various studies have shown that students whose intention was to understand the meaning of what they were reading tended to work by deep processing, while those whose style was strategic processing had planned their work to acquire only those facts they thought would be needed to pass the examinations.

A number of educationists have developed this understanding of the way students learn. In Southampton, Coles (1990) investigated medical students and found that the most successful students (as judged by examinations) used what he termed an elaborated approach to learning, which he saw as one type of deep processing. These students were able to integrate their earlier preclinical learning with more recent clinical work, discovering interrelationships between the different subjects especially during revision. They were then able to fit them together and reflect on the significance of the connections they were making. Elaboration is the drawing of multiple and complex links between items of knowledge. This has been linked to the work of a number of investigators such as Norman (1988) who have suggested that successful clinical reasoning is dependent on access to a memory story of deep, rich, and elaborated conceptual knowledge. Students will become better problem-solvers through an educational strategy that enhances their ability to seek out and make multiple links in their learning, reflecting on the significance of these. Two instructional approaches that are of importance here are problem-based learning (PBL) and the concept of reflection.

Problem-based learning

Problem-based learning has been fully described elsewhere by Barrows and Tamblyn (1980). In this approach, the student takes on a patient problem, a health-delivery problem, or a research problem as a stimulus for learning in areas considered appropriate by the student at that time. Problem-based learning has been the basis of educational strategies in many of the newer innovative medical schools such as the University of Limburg at Maastricht, or the University of McMaster, Ontario. Norman (1988) differentiated between learning problem-solving skills and learning through the use of problems. He considered that attempts to instil certain clinical reasoning and problem-solving skills were questionable, but that the use of problem-based learning as an educational strategy to increase conceptual knowledge was well-proven. PBL has been extensively reviewed by Walton and Matthews (1989), and the theoretical premises have been set out by Schmidt (1993) who considered there were five important cognitive effects:

(1) Activation of prior knowledge through the initial analysis of a problem.
(2) Elaboration on prior knowledge and active processing of new information through small-group discussion.
(3) Restructuring of knowledge in order to fit the problem presented.
(4) Contextual learning with the problem serving as a scaffold for storing cues that may support retrieval of relevant knowledge when needed for similar problems.
(5) The emergence of epistemic curiosity as students tend to see the relevance of problems.

Problem-based learning provides both relevance and linkage to previously acquired knowledge. In form it is exactly what it states. It is an educational approach in which students tackle problems in small groups, usually under the supervision of a tutor. The problems may be presented in a variety of ways: on paper, on film, through pathological specimens, or through real patients. People constantly learn by solving problems, often in a haphazard way. The key to designing a problem-based programme is to ensure that the materials trigger learning objectives that are appropriate to the course or session. Many courses are now using PBL methods and descriptions will be found in the References (see David and Patel 1995; Engel 1992). The method is described further in Chapter 14.

Reflection

Reflection is a key theme in another salient perspective on professional education and development provided in Schön's seminal book *Educating the reflective practitioner* (Schön 1987). Starting from the premise that, in those activities or professions which combine academic learning with practical work, certain individuals are identifiably more excellent than the majority, Schön set out to find what characterized those practitioners. He found, through a large series of empirical studies, that these were people who consistently *reflected* on their work, in such a way that they continually learned from it. This model, of *the reflective practitioner*, seems to represent an ideal for any doctor, and therefore an appropriate aim for medical education. A central component of educating the reflective practitioner is treating the student as an adult, and allowing him or her to discover *how to learn*. Awareness of this educational research can help us understand students. Consider these questions:

- Do tutors seek to discover what is currently motivating students?
- Students will often use strategic processing in view of the pressure of assessments. How adequate is this?
- How can students be helped to be reflective, discover links, and elaborate their knowledge?

THE FRAMEWORK FOR EDUCATION: THE CURRICULUM

Learning, even self-learning, has to take place within some framework. A curriculum is a description of the structure of a course, an outline of the arrangement of its component parts. It contrasts with a syllabus which is just a summary list of the topics or subjects studied on a course, a sort of bill of fare or menu. Sometimes, a differentiation is made between the *official* curriculum set by the faculty, the *hidden* curriculum which is determined by the areas that are assessed and examined (i.e. what the faculty demonstrates as important) and the *real* curriculum which is what students actually study. Frequently, the real curriculum is determined more by the hidden than the official curriculum. The aim should be to make the official, hidden, and real curricula synonymous so that students find the framework for learning appropriate to their needs. This is discussed further in Part V. This chapter is concerned with the structure of the official curriculum and the way it provides a framework for learning.

Undergraduate medical education can take the form of a number of different curriculum types (which are not mutually exclusive):

- two-stage;
- vertically integrated;
- horizontally integrated;
- spiral.

The two-stage curriculum (Fig. 2.1)

This has been the traditional pattern in many countries. Indeed, in the past it might have been considered a three-stage course, for there was a 'premedical' stage of physics, chemistry, and biology. Most students now cover these at school in attaining A levels, HSC, or equivalent, but some universities still provide a premedical course for students who have a background in the humanities.

Typically, the two-stage curriculum comprises a preclinical course that covers the basic sciences of anatomy, physiology, and biochemistry. Recently, behavioural sciences such as sociology and psychology have been included and some courses also embrace pharmacology and microbiology at this stage. This is followed by a clinical course where medical skills are learnt within clinical disciplines and pathological science is taught. There is often no contact between the two parts, which may be taught in different places (university campus and hospital).

Within each section of the course, subjects are clearly separated by discipline.

Physiology, biochemistry, and anatomy or medicine, surgery, and paediatrics all have their allotted hours and are all assessed separately. It is usually necessary to satisfy the preclinical examiners before the student is allowed to proceed to clinical work.

Although this traditional pattern will be familiar to many readers, the rigid two-stage course is now becoming a thing of the past in most UK medical schools.

Vertically integrated curricula (Fig. 2.2)

This term implies that components which have been taught sequentially in a traditional curriculum are, instead, taught together. For example, consider the nervous system. In a two-stage course the anatomy and physiology of the nervous system are taught in preclinical years, although at different times. Only in the clinical years will students be taught about the symptoms, signs, pathology, and management of patients with neurological disease. In a vertically integrated course the anatomy and physiology of the nervous system will be learnt concurrently with neuropathology, neurology, neurosurgery, and other relevant aspects of clinical medicine. However, the learning will take place in different and separate settings such as dissecting rooms, lecture theatres, medical and surgical wards, and laboratories; each discipline may continue to teach according to their own subcurricula.

Horizontally integrated curricula (Fig. 2.3)

Horizontal integration means that at any stage of the course the boundaries between disciplines is blurred. In the example of the nervous system, teachers from anatomy,

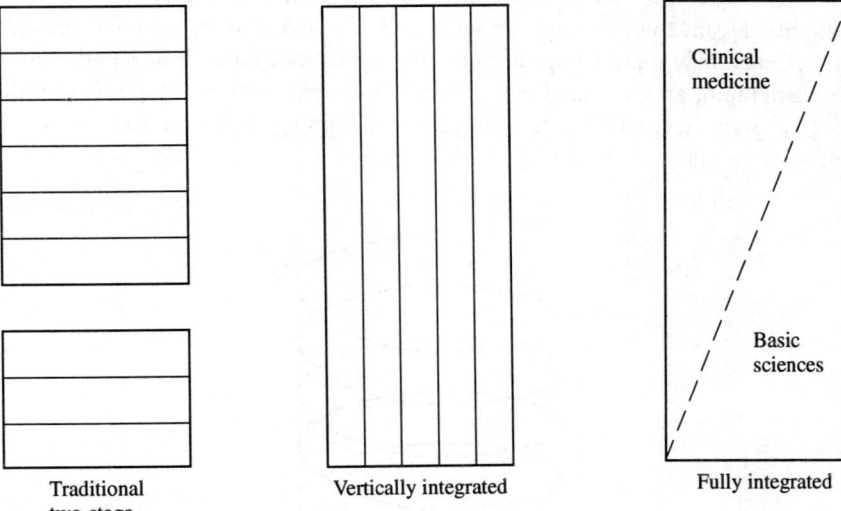

Traditional two-stage	Vertically integrated	Fully integrated

Fig 2.1 The two-stage curriculum.

Fig 2.2 A vertically integrated curriculum.

Fig 2.3 A horizontally integrated curriculum.

physiology, pathology, and the clinical disciplines would work together to provide a single course in 'nerves and their diseases'. This requires greater collaboration between teachers than with vertical integration. This is shown pictorially by the broken line between basic sciences and clinical medicine in Fig. 2.3.

Of course, vertical and horizontal integration can be combined. Fully integrated courses are often systems-based where students work on a whole system (such as the respiratory system) using the resources of both the basic and clinical sciences to learn about the normal behaviour and the diseases of that system.

Problem-based learning (see above) provides a further development of full integration. From the starting point of a specific clinical problem students seek information, skills, and practical experience in all relevant fields, drawing on the full range of learning resources. Because of the nature of clinical problems these will ensure that the broader aspects of psychological and social issues are included.

The spiral curriculum (Fig. 2.4)

When such a course also provides for iterative revisiting of subjects throughout the course it is described as spiral. The value of a spiral lies in its property of reinforcement: a behaviour, a concept, or a value once learned is reinforced if it is revisited in a way that gives positive feedback. A student who discovers that using a simple skill (such as asking open questions) leads to high-quality information being elicited, will go on using that skill. A piece of knowledge gained early in the course on, say, alcohol abuse, which is retrieved and applied at a later stage (when the curriculum spirals back to alcohol problems) will be reinforced, and the knowledge deepened. In terms of Bloom's (1985) hierarchy this enables factual recall to advance to understanding and synthesis.

The theoretical basis for an integrated curriculum lies in the ideas of grounding learning in relevant contexts, and explicitly building new learning on prior knowledge. Instead of each new topic being discrete, often unconnected with those adjacent to it in the curriculum, an integrated curriculum means that each new topic is introduced in a logical sequence, which relates to previous learning, has a relevant context, and is conducive to elaborated learning (Coles 1990).

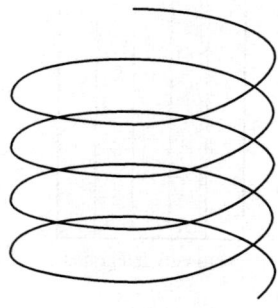

Fig 2.4   A spiral curriculum.

Core and options

There is a further consideration in looking at curriculum, especially in considering the problems of information overload. Although it is clear that there are certain knowledge, skills, and attitudes that any basic doctor requires, it is also true that different students may have particular interests and abilities and these need to be developed as well if the curriculum is to be truly learner-centred. This has led to the concept of a 'core and options' curriculum. It is now recommended that a considerable part of the course should be devoted to allowing students to pursue in breadth or depth areas of personal interest (known originally as options and now as special study modules). This has also meant that medical schools have had to work at defining the core curriculum on which every student will be assessed. In the Netherlands this has been done centrally with the provision of a document (*Blueprint 1994*) which all medical schools have agreed to follow (Metz *et al*. 1994). In the United Kingdom individual schools have been allowed to develop their own core content, although there will clearly be a considerable degree of agreement on these.

Further questions

Some questions about developing a curriculum remain. Consider these:

- What advantages of the traditional two-stage course have enabled it to survive so long?
- How well do tutors from different disciplines work together in facilitating an integrated curriculum?
- What determines the areas of learning students concentrate on?
- What places do students perceives as relevant contexts for their learning (i.e. where do they prefer to learn)?
- What are the difficulties in setting a core curriculum?

CONCLUSION

Contemporary education is concerned about having clear and measurable objectives, and about making the optimal use of the student's learning abilities to achieve these. Designing a course, especially in a field of burgeoning knowledge such as medicine, requires that both these factors are taken into account. In the past there was too much emphasis on adding new objectives without consideration of whether these could be effectively achieved in the time available. The result was often a concentration on the knowledge base with insufficient consideration of wider objectives in other domains. Integrated courses with a focus on the core content are beginning to address this issue. Those seeking to develop community-oriented education must be aware of this and not fall into the traps of the past.

3 Objectives of undergraduate medical education

The overall aim of undergraduate medical education derived from the General Medical Council (1993) recommendations can be summarized as:

To produce a caring doctor competent to deliver the highest quality of health care, able to advance the science of medicine and eager to go on learning more.

With this aim in mind each medical school will have general educational goals and objectives for its whole curriculum from which more specific objectives will be constructed for different units of teaching. These will differ depending on the curriculum and the different levels of integration.

Table 3.1, which appears as an appendix to this chapter, reproduces the goals and objectives published by the Education Committee of the General Medical Council (GMC 1993) as guidelines for British undergraduate medical education. They are subdivided into the three domains of learning – knowledge (cognitive), skills (psychomotor), and attitudes (affective).

It has been customary for the GMC to express its guidance to medical schools in the form of such a list of objectives. These are not intended to be prescriptive but rather formative, to be adapted by each school according to its own resources and educational ethos. They are set in very general terms and might be considered to lack sufficient explicitness. Such generalizations as 'the student will have acquired a knowledge and understanding of . . . the sciences basic to medicine' are, however, to be expected at a course level. They need to be defined more rigidly when individual teaching blocks and units are considered. It is important to remember to differentiate between broad course objectives and defined educational objectives for specific learning programmes. A list, such as that provided by the GMC, does not formally determine which objectives should be achieved in the context of the community. All these objectives will be achieved through learning in many different settings, especially in an integrated course. However, it is possible to see how experience in the community can contribute to realizing these goals and objectives and so to set more specific objectives for learning in that context including the fields of general practice and primary health care.

The remainder of this chapter provides a general overview of setting objectives within this context. The next chapter provides greater detail for a range of objectives, presented under 10 headings, for which the community is a potential setting for learning.

KNOWLEDGE OBJECTIVES

Knowledge can be acquired by reading books or articles, watching videos and listening to lectures but, unless the information is applied in some way, it is unlikely to be remembered. Knowledge is applied when it is synthesized into some new form (such as writing an essay), or used in a group discussion. Better still, knowledge is applied when it is used to solve a problem, either real or simulated. With this in mind a number of objectives relating to acquisition and application of knowledge could be set for learning in the community.

Assuming suitable sources of information are available to the student, such as access to libraries, computers and audio-visual resources, students could achieve objectives relating to an understanding of how people react to illness (1(d))* and a knowledge and understanding of human relationships (1(i)). Similarly, an understanding of environmental and social determinants of disease, the burden of disease within the community, and principles of disease prevention and health promotion (1(e),(f)) represent Public Health objectives, which could be learned entirely from a community base (not necessarily in general practice, but using the resources of Health Authorities or their equivalents).

Understanding disease processes (1(c)), clearly requires some learning in appropriate laboratory settings, but this has to be linked to clinical presentation and achieving objectives related to the range of problems, solutions, and principles of therapy (1(b),(g)) requires experience in community as well as hospital settings.

Understanding human relationships, including the special field of reproduction (1(h)) and the importance of communication (1(j)), the organization, management, and provision of health care (1(1)), and the ethical and legal issues relevant to medical practice (1(k)) are all areas where objectives can be set and achieved within the community. It is clear that this particular setting can contribute to the achievement of all the main knowledge objectives.

SKILLS OBJECTIVES

There is no doubt that basic clinical skills (2(a)) can be acquired outside hospital, provided competent teachers are available and there is enough time. Ophthalmoscopy, for instance, can be taught in the community. It is true that organizing rapid experience of a range of conditions may prove easier in a ward where many patients with eye problems are concentrated but, with a suitable length of attachment, similar experience can be achieved in the community.

Skills objectives concerned with many basic clinical procedures (2(b)), such as inserting an intravenous line, are more suitable for a hospital setting. However, there are other procedures in which proficiency needs to be gained at some time, from syringing ears for wax to injecting joints, which are increasingly performed in general practice. If

---

* Throughout the remainder of this chapter the figures in brackets relate to the GMC (1993) objectives in Table 3.1 (p. 37–39).

such procedures are included in the specific objectives of the medical school, they could be learnt by students in the community under appropriately supervised conditions.

General practice is now well established in its use of computerized information systems during patient contact. The community is therefore an ideal setting for students to learn some of the basic information skills of handling computer systems and build on experience gained in other settings (2(c)).

ATTITUDINAL OBJECTIVES

All the attitudinal objectives (3 (a–l)) can be addressed within the community. For some of them this setting provides a particular interest and bent.

General practitioner trainers are used to considering patient-centred attitudes (3(a),(b),(f)). Sometimes, registrars in general practice, coming from a series of junior hospital posts where the emphasis was mainly on biomedical aspects of patient care (clerking patients, getting the right tests done, dealing with medical emergencies), actually need to relearn them.

The ability to cope with uncertainty (3(d)) is a major requirement in a situation where people present with unstructured illness. The ethical conflicts implied in developing an awareness of the moral responsibilities involved in individual patient care *and* the provision of care to populations (3(e)) are well known to practitioners in the community. Students will also obtain different insights from exposure to teachers in the community who are involved in self-audit (3(g)) and the advancement of medical knowledge (3(l)).

THE SETTING OF OBJECTIVES

The goals and broad objectives have usually been set by those responsible for a course, taking on board the recommendations of an organization, such as the GMC, and other indications of public demand. Traditionally, this may have been done by a curriculum committee or a particular department or other provider. This clearly provides some control over the overall direction of the learning. However, these general objectives have to be considered in the light of the needs of the group of learners with their particular strengths and weaknesses. Designers of course modules and individual tutors have to develop a programme of learning in the light of these considerations and so define more detailed educational objectives. Learners, as well as individual tutors, have an important role in this, especially for short courses or individual sessions.

Objectives set by students

Can students decide on their own objectives? Self-set objectives would appear to have two advantages over imposed objectives: they are *owned* by the learner, and therefore have greater salience, and they are perceived to be *achievable*, and might be expected to be more often achieved. Their disadvantages arise from the lack of control by the department of faculty, and the variation between students, making objective-based assessment less easy.

These problems can be overcome by providing overall general objectives and inviting students to define their personal, more specific, objectives based on their perceived learning needs. Stanley and Al-Shehri (1992) reported the experience of one medical school where the general practice course required students to set their own objectives. The 110 self-set objectives could be classified into 10 categories:

(1) consolidating existing knowledge;
(2) epidemiology (including social and psychological factors in illness);
(3) the role of the GP (including service provision, ethical issues);
(4) the work of general practice (prevention and health promotion);
(5) the clinical interview (communication skills);
(6) physical examination (consolidating, and acquiring new skills);
(7) problem handling (prescribing, referral to specialists, management of common conditions);
(8) understanding roles (primary care teams, primary-secondary interface);
(9) management in general practice (organization, finance, computers, contracts);
(10) general practice as a career option (do I want to do it?).

What is interesting about this list is what was omitted: there is no apparent mention of attitudes. This suggests that students are not particularly aware of the need to think about or change these. The question arises what happens when students do not pick up major objectives of the course.

The students in Stanley and Al-Shehri's study were following a traditional course, in which most of the teaching had been didactic, but where general practice was trying to inject an element of learner-centredness through the self-set objectives. As a result, the students' vision of what could be learnt on a course might have been limited by their previous experience. Had this been part of a problem-based course, the objectives might have been different. One of the great benefits of problem-based learning is that it requires students to think for themselves about what they need to learn. This takes place in the controlled setting of a tutorial group. The role of the tutor in such a group is to ensure that the essential elements of the module are being addressed without being too directive. Therefore if, as is very likely, there are attitudinal objectives set for a module, the group tutor might, if the group does not discover them for itself, point this fact out to the group during the discussions. The group would then have an opportunity to reconsider its objectives.

Objectives set between tutor and student

Time spent in a discipline such as general practice offers special opportunities in the undergraduate course for the student to develop a one-to-one relationship with a tutor. Depending on the structure of the course, the student can spend a considerable amount of time with an individual tutor. This may be concentrated, for example, over a four-week module, or intermittent contact may be provided over a much longer period of the course. In either case, the one-to-one relationship between a tutor and student offers opportunities to identify strengths and weaknesses and so consider the individual learning needs of students. These can be defined as specific educational objectives and addressed as opportunities arise.

The personal objectives should relate to the overall course objectives, but the types of learning experience chosen to achieve them may differ markedly from student to student. This is partly because of the variety of resources available to meet those needs, which will vary from setting to setting and from one period in time to another. The tutor should try to identify a student's learning needs at the start of a module or period of contact asking them to set their own objectives. Students will vary considerably in their ability to identify their own learning needs, depending particularly on their previous exposure to adult learning methods. If the concept of self-set objectives is unfamiliar they can be asked:

- what they are hoping to gain from the course;
- whether there are particular things they wish to learn;
- whether they have identified areas of weakness which they would like to address.

In helping to identify knowledge objectives, the tutor needs to know what stage in the course each student is at. In many courses learning in a general practice setting forms part of a rotation of 'specialty' subjects, and future experiences may need to be related to what the student has done in the past. Students should be able identify specific skills which they need to acquire or practice, and which are appropriate to community settings.

The tutor should draw a distinction between student-identified objectives, whether needs or wants, and needs the tutor identifies in relation to the course objectives. Where there is a discrepancy between these, an explicit discussion with the student will prevent frustration if the range of experiences offered does not appear to match the student's self-set objectives especially in the domain of attitudes where needs are more likely to be detected by the tutor than offered by students. The course objectives defined by the medical school can be discussed individually with students. This helps to put their experience into context, and enables a framework to be developed for the various experiences to which students will be exposed during an individual module.

Learning needs may be identified with the student at the start of a module, but may also become apparent during the course of time spent with the tutor. Tutors may become aware that students are stronger in an area than they had previously perceived, or some hidden weakness may become apparent. Identification of such weaknesses may lead to the definition of further learning objectives for the module, and to revision of the planned experience to meet the identified needs.

In the general practice setting consulting sessions provide an important opportunity to identify student strength and weaknesses. This will in general require that the student does more than sit, watch, and discuss cases. It is important for the tutor to be able to observe students both talking to and examining patients to identify problems with examination and communication skills, as well as identifying inappropriate attitudes. The attitudinal problems which are most likely to surface are a lack of respect for patients and for other members of the primary health care team. Lack of respect for patients may be manifest as an inability to appreciate that the patients' concerns and expectations are an important and legitimate part of the consultation, but can also be revealed by a clumsy and insensitive approach to physical examination. Identification of inappropriate attitudes to others members of the primary care team is an important part of community attachments, and is one reason why a tutor should obtain brief feedback from all members of the primary care team to whom a student is attached.

Tutors in general practice often have the opportunity and ability to identify and negotiate individual learning needs and objectives with students. They may also have the opportunity to build up a strong enough relationship to show students that what they think they want is not always what they need. Students commonly want to do things in areas in which they already have considerable strengths. They can be encouraged by having these strengths reinforced and then directed towards other needs. Sometimes for the first time, a tutor is able to seriously address what a student's individual needs are. This opportunity within general practice is often one reason for students giving high positive feedback about community attachments.

Individuals with problems

Although not specifically concerned with objective-setting, there is no doubt that as tutors and students work together to look at educational needs individual problems will be identified. The closeness of the relationship between tutor and student in a one-to-one attachment may mean that the tutor is in an unusually good position to identify major problems which the student faces. These may be major psychosocial problems or doubts about continuing medicine. When this happens it may provide an opportunity for students to have confidential discussions about their problems outside the more formal academic structure. It has been the experience of many GP tutors that the tutor/ counsellor role sometimes becomes blurred, even within an attachment lasting only a few weeks. Although such experiences can often be put to the student's advantage, tutors need to be careful to avoid conflicts of interest between teaching and counselling roles, especially if the former involves the tutor in summative assessment which may influence the student's career.

Setting objectives for individual sessions

When objectives are set for a module or a specific week, individual sessions and surgeries will consist of tasks that help to achieve those objectives. If the objective relates to learning the indications for prescribing antibiotics, students might be given tasks to consider the appropriateness of each prescription issued. However, objectives can also be defined for individual sessions or even surgeries. Such sessional objectives should relate to the overall objectives of the attachment and the educational purpose of other aspects such as seminar or project work. They may make use of the student's unusual status as observer on a one-to-one consultation. Possible objectives for individual consulting sessions could include learning the variety of presentations in general practice or the factors involved in a triaxial (clinical, personal, and contextual) diagnosis. Considering possible objectives helps to set tasks for the students while they are sitting in the consultation and can help to stimulate the uncommunicative student.

They can also be helpful in focusing the thoughts of occasional students who are overwhelmed by the diversity of problems seen in a general practice setting, and may find an anchor of a limited objective helpful for the way in which they learn during a consulting session.

Sessional objectives can also be set for other experiences in the community such as those arranged within the primary care team. For example, attachment with the district nurse can be set in the context of providing continuing care for patients with chronic illness, and also in the context of understanding how different members of the primary care team relate to one another and how their individual roles need to be valued within the team. Setting experience in the context of specific objectives also helps the tutor to 'debrief' on individual experiences. Rather than just saying: 'How did you get on with the district nurse?' they can ask the student to describe the role of a nurse in the management of a specific disease.

So far, approaches to setting objectives for time spent in a community setting have been addressed in terms of a model where general practice offers defined courses within the medical curriculum. This reflects the current situation in most medical schools. However, many schools are moving rapidly towards integrated curricula. In these courses the objectives of community sessions will need to be tied much more closely to the parts of the course with which they integrate. Tutors will need to become more aware than they are at present of the overall course objectives and educational experience. Students will often arrive with clear objectives and will request tasks that achieve that purpose.

CONCLUSION

This chapter has sought to develop the concept of educational objectives and discuss how students can be encouraged to set and work with precise, short-term objectives as they proceed through the course.

The three domains of learning (cognitive, psychomotor, and affective) have been applied to the medical course, and related to the community. As undergraduate teaching moves more into the community, it is essential that all those who aspire to teach or learning recognize the whole spectrum of learning, and understand the function of explicit learning objectives in guiding learning and in shaping assessment. In the next chapter a number of specific objectives are discussed in greater detail.

Readers may wish at this point to ask themselves these questions:

• What are the objectives of the course or block that the students are undertaking?
• Which objectives are achievable within a community setting such as general practice?
• Is there a balance between knowledge, skills, and attitudes in the objectives set for a block (or a session)?
• Is there a clear process to follow if students have difficulty: (a)–in negotiating objectives? (b)–in achieving objectives?

Appendix. Table 3.1 Goals and objectives of undergraduate medical education (from GMC 1993)

GOALS

(a) The student should acquire a KNOWLEDGE and UNDERSTANDING of health and its promotion, and of disease, its prevention and management, in the context of the whole individual and his or her place in the family and in society.

(b) The student should acquire and become proficient in basic clinical SKILLS, such as the ability to obtain a patient's history, to undertake a comprehensive physical and mental state examination and interpret the findings, and to demonstrate competence in the performance of a limited number of basic technical procedures.

(c) The student should acquire and demonstrate ATTITUDES necessary for the achievement of high standards of medical practice, both in relation to the provision of care of individuals and populations and to his or her own personal development.

OBJECTIVES
1. Knowledge objectives

At the end of the undergraduate course the student will have acquired a knowledge and understanding of:

(a) the *sciences basic to medicine*, and
- (i) the discovery of how knowledge is acquired,
- (ii) an understanding of research methods,
- (iii) an ability to evaluate evidence.

(b) the *range of problems* that are presented to doctors and the *range of solutions* that have been developed for their recognition, investigation, prevention, and treatment;

(c) *diseases* in terms of *processes*, both mental and physical, such as trauma, inflammation, immune response, degeneration, neoplasia, metabolic disturbance, and genetic disorder;

(d) how *disease presents* in patients of all ages, how patients react to illness or to the belief that they are ill, and how illness behaviour varies between social and cultural groups;

(e) the *environmental and social determinants* of disease, the principles of disease surveillance and the means by which diseases may spread, and the analysis of the burden of disease within the community;

(f) the principles of *disease prevention and health promotion*;

(g) the principles of *therapy*, including:
- (i) the management of acute illness;
- (ii) the actions of drugs, their prescription, and administration;
- (iii) the care of the chronically ill and the disabled;
- (iv) rehabilitation, institutional, and community care;
- (v) the amelioration of suffering and the relief of pain;
- (vi) the care of the dying;

(h) *reproduction*, including:

    (i)   pregnancy and childbirth;
    (ii) fertility and contraception;
    (iii) psychological aspects;
(i)   *human relationships*, individual and community;
(j)   the importance of *communication*, both with patients and their relatives and with other professionals, both medical and non-medical, involved in their care;
(k)   ethical and legal issues relevant to the practice of medicine;
(l)   the *organization, management, and provision of health care*, both in the community and in hospital, the economic and practical constraints within which it is delivered, and the audit process to monitor its delivery.

2. *Skills objectives*

At the end of the course of undergraduate education the student will have acquired and will have demonstrated his or her proficiency in communication and the other essential skills of medicine, including:

(a) *basic clinical methods*, including the ability to:
    (i)   obtain and record a comprehensive history;
    (ii) perform a complete physical examination, and assess the mental state;
    (iii) interpret the findings obtained from the history and the physical examination;
    (iv) reach a provisional assessment of patients' problems and formulate with them plans for investigation and management.

(b) *basic clinical procedures* including:
    (i)   Basic and Advanced Life Support;
    (ii) venepuncture;
    (iii) insertion of an intravenous line.

[The guidelines indicate that there are many more procedures in which doctors need to gain proficiency, but that the precise stage of their training that each is learned will vary from school to school: it is important that medical schools consult with Postgraduate Deans and higher training bodies in compiling a list of procedures which will be covered in the undergraduate course.]

(c) *basic computing skills* as applied to medicine.

3. *Attitudinal objectives*

At the end of the course of undergraduate medical education the student will have acquired and will demonstrate attitudes essential to the practice of medicine, including:

(a) respect for patients and colleagues that encompasses, without prejudice, diversity of background and opportunity, language, culture, and way of life;
(b) the recognition of patients' rights in all respects, and particularly in regard to confidentiality and informed consent;
(c) approaches to learning that are based on curiosity and the exploration of knowledge rather than on its passive acquisition, and that will be retained throughout professional life;

(d) the ability to cope with uncertainty;

(e) awareness of the moral and ethical responsibilities involved in individual patient care and in the provision of care to populations of patients; such awareness must be developed early in the course;

(f) awareness of the need to ensure that the highest possible quality of patient care must always be provided;

(g) development of the capacity for self-audit and for participation in the peer review process;

(h) awareness of personal limitations, a willingness to seek help when necessary, and ability to work effectively as a member of a team;

(i) willingness to use his or her professional capabilities to contribute to community as well as to individual patient welfare by the practice of preventive medicine and the encouragement of health promotion;

(j) ability to adapt to change;

(k) awareness of the need for continuing professional development allied to the process of continuing medical education, in order to ensure that high levels of clinical competence and knowledge are maintained;

(l) acceptance of the responsibility to contribute as far as possible to the advancement of medical knowledge in order to benefit medical practice and further improve the quality of patient care.

4 Learning objectives for the community

Educational objectives in nine areas, particularly relevant to learning in community settings such as general practice, are now discussed. A tenth part addresses the attitudinal objectives, since these can be considered generic, in the sense that they can apply across all settings.

Each section provides some sample objectives. These are not intended to be an exhaustive list as this would belie the basic principles of learner-centredness and self-direction. They also lack a time element although normally they would be prefaced by a statement such as 'At the end of an attachment, (or module or course) . . .' Educators should work out precise objectives for their own settings, ideally in collaboration with the learners.

1. LEARNING ABOUT THE COMMUNITY (GMC Objective 1(e))*

Many of these objectives derive from the population perspective of public health medicine. This addresses the distribution of people and disease in communities (the sciences of demography and epidemiology). It also considers the assessment of and provision for health needs, in the statutory, private, and voluntary sectors. As well as these factual and quantitative aspects students need to learn about communities from a qualitative viewpoint. They should be able to describe communities in the light of social, environmental, cultural, and anthropological factors.

Students need to understand how populations are described, in terms of age, sex, and other demographic variables. One example would be how the relative deprivation of a population is measured. The use of the Jarman Index, or a similar measure, would enable this to be taught using data from a single general practice or neighbourhood. Students also need to learn from the wider perspective of public health and the analysis of the areas covered by health commissions.

Mortality and morbidity are described by rates. Students need to know how a standardized mortality ratio (SMR) is derived with the rate standardized to a common population, usually the National population, and converted to a ratio. They also need to learn how a concept such as the SMR for a given cause of death or a morbidity rate can be applied in assessing the needs of populations of different sizes including an individual practice.

---

* Figures in brackets refer to the list of GMC objectives in Tabel 3.1 (p. 37–39).

Students can also learn to evaluate the source of such statistics. Some of these sources, such as death certificates, are very unreliable. Within a general practice students can discover the problems of writing such certificates or of using diagnostic labels in morbidity recording. The validation of, for example, cancer registry data, can be addressed by discovering the way general practitioners are involved in the process of follow-up by certain disease registries.

Lastly, students can learn how to obtain qualitative date about a community or a group of people with a disabling condition by devising and using a questionnaire on a sample of a practice or district population.

Sample objectives

The student should be able to:

- describe a range of environmental factors that influence health;
- describe a population in terms of its social and cultural features;
- estimate the expected patterns of illness from age—sex histograms of district or practice populations and appropriate SMR data;
- Use data provided by a single general practice, derive crude morbidity rates for common chronic diseases, and explain their limitations;
- design and use a questionnaire to explore one aspect of lifestyle in a sample population;
- explore, describe, and evaluate the provision of health care for a major chronic disease.

2. LEARNING ABOUT THE FAMILY (GMC Objectives 1(h), (i))

In primary care, family medicine is an alternative name for general practice used by many countries, and general practitioners are often referred to as family doctors. Health visitors may also be known as family visitors. Primary care is therefore a good setting to consider objectives relating to the family.

Families may be considered as very small communities or groups. They can therefore enable students to learn about sociopsychological factors affecting health, illness, and health care. Students need to grasp the importance of understanding the immediate social contexts of patients. This requires understanding of the concept of a family which can be considered from social, psychological, and genetic perspectives.

Social

The constructs of social support systems such as families have major influences on health, and how people respond to illness. Students need to be able to describe these and to define expressions such as:

- *Nuclear family*: members of one or two generations living together (i.e. parent(s) and their children).

- *Extended family*: a wider range of relationships linked by blood or adoption, and including other generations, and wider relationships, whether living together or not.
- *Household*: those living under one roof, inclusive of non-kin, such as lodgers, or simply an informal group of individuals, such as students sharing a flat.

At every level of illness, it is normally these social support systems, and especially families, who provide care. This is particularly true for the bulk of care for the elderly and disabled. This role has recently been recognized by the state benefits system, with the introduction of an Invalid Care Allowance. This means that relatives and carers can also require information and support.

Psychological

Families also affect the emotional development of patients, especially children. Students need to discover the normal stages of development, be able to identify the range of normal behaviours, and know the important signs of problems (especially various forms of child abuse). At the other end of the life cycle, families are situations where the most intense grief may be experienced when one member dies. Bereavement is best understood in the context of the family and the community, rather than in the more strained atmosphere of a hospital.

Relationships within a family frequently contribute to the causes of mental illness. These relationships are in turn influenced by the health of family members. Students need to have a basic understanding of such family dynamics, although in the past undergraduate medical education in the United Kingdom has not paid great attention to an area often seen as a postgraduate topic.

Genetic

The third family perspective to consider is genetics, where inherited disease is the prime concern. This is an area of increasing importance. Many diseases are recognized to have a genetic component (e.g. ischaemic heart disease, type II diabetes, and various forms of arthritis), while single-gene diseases (such as cystic fibrosis, sickle-cell anaemia and thalassaemia) assume great importance for those families in which they occur. Students should recognize the value of carefully documenting family history of such diseases, and of exploring, with the patient, their understanding of the implications of such a history.

These different perspectives give an entirely new meaning to the concept of a family history. Students need to learn that both present and past members of a family may have great significance for other members, whether in social, psychological, or genetic terms. A range of objectives can be considered as students have increasing contacts with families and households.

Sample objectives

The student should be able to:

- describe a range of households and family structures and state the implications of each;
- take a family history from a patient, including psychological and social components;
- describe and chart the relationships between the members of a given family, and apply this information to a presented problem;
- construct a family tree (genogram) for a family with an inherited (genetic) condition;
- talk empathically with a bereaved person;
- recognize a dysfunctional family, and explain some of the mechanisms which might cause the dysfunction.

3. LEARNING ABOUT THE INDIVIDUAL (GMC Objectives 1(d), (j), (k))

The essential component of medical practice is the occasion when, in the intimacy of the consulting room, a person who is ill, or who believes himself to be ill, seeks the advice of a doctor whom he trusts. This is a consultation, and all else in the practice of medicine derives from it. (Spence 1960)

Spence's oft-quoted aphorism probably overemphasizes the individual consultation, but for many doctors it is the central activity, on which all else depends. Students in a community setting have the opportunity of spending time with individual patients without the distractions often found in a hospital ward, or the focused programme of many out-patient clinics. In this situation they can develop their communication skills with individuals. They can also, by using appropriate listening skills, find out a great deal about an individual from which they can learn more general principles of illness behaviour, communication, and ethics.

They can learn about reasons for attendance. Patients consult their GP for different sorts of reasons:

- their tolerance of a symptom may have reached its limit;
- their anxiety about a symptom may have exceeded a threshold (students need to know how this differs from the first);
- the doctor may have invited them (e.g. for follow-up, immunization, or screening);
- they may have an administrative need (e.g. a medical certificate);
- they may consult about another person: a relative or friend.

Students can learn different models of illness. The traditional biomedical model of illness considered a patient to be made up of body systems, within which are organs, tissues, cells, organelles, molecules, and atoms. Disease is malfunction at one of these levels, and treatment is directed accordingly. In the biopsychosocial model, a person is seen in a far wider context. There are the micro levels of molecule, cell, tissue, but there are levels beyond the individual such as family, social group, and society. Illness can be identified as malfunction at these levels as well as at the cellular level. Thus, a heart attack can be seen to affect not only the myocardium, but also the person's self-esteem, place in the family as bread-winner, and function in society. There is also a time element: individuals change and develop and students need to learn how this affects people (Engel 1980).

Sample objectives

The student should be able to:

- achieve an effective rapport with patients of all ages, and either sex;
- conduct an interview in order to gather a comprehensive account of a patient's problem(s), their perceptions of health, and their feelings;
- monitor the process of a consultation and show how they might modify their behaviour accordingly;
- value the patient's view of their reasons for consultation, aware that an effective solution needs to take account of these;
- describe the normal processes of development, through infancy, childhood, adolescence, adulthood, and ageing;
- calibrate a patient's level of functioning in order to use appropriate language and ideas.

4. LEARNING ABOUT HEALTH AND ITS PROMOTION (GMC Objective 1(f))

People normally function within their communities. This setting is therefore the appropriate one for learning about the concept of health. Health is clearly more than the absence of disease but students need to be able to explore different definitions and see how they can be applied. The World Health Organization definition of health as a state of complete physical, mental, and spiritual well-being, sounds all-embracing. On reflection it may be considered impractical because it is probably impossible to achieve, or to measure. Other definitions refer to individuals fulfilling their potential, or achieving their optimum performance. Thus a person who has lost both legs in an accident, but who has just won the world championship 400-metres race in a wheelchair could reasonably be described as healthy. Such examples can demonstrate important distinctions between impairment, disability, and handicap and show that health is about functioning, and the perception of well-being, rather than primarily about disease.

From considering definitions, students need to learn about the measurement of health, which is both complex and multidimensional. They also need to consider how behaviour influences health in both positive and negative ways, and the way that disease affects health. This will lead to developing objectives concerned with promotion of health. Community-based learning allows students access to people and groups who are healthy in a range of situations from schools and residential homes for the elderly to well-person and other screening clinics. Health promotion can be observed in context, making it possible to learn concepts of primary, secondary, and tertiary prevention.

Sample objectives

Students should be able to:

- identify risk-taking behaviours in patients, and discuss them in the context of health promotion;
- distinguish between primary, secondary, and tertiary prevention of disease;
- distinguish between impairment, disability and handicap, and understand the relationship between them;
- describe at least one commonly used health status assessment instrument;
- describe and apply a simple strategy for smoking cessation.

5. LEARNING ABOUT ILLNESS, DISEASE, AND DISABILITY
(GMC Objectives 1(b), (c))

The majority of illness episodes are managed entirely in primary care, but clearly it is the more serious or the more rare presentations that are referred to hospitals. With the advent of a core curriculum medical students could encounter most of the key problems through experience outside hospitals. Important exceptions are major trauma and, in urban areas, acute medical emergencies where patients are taken immediately to hospital. It is also true that many treatments can only be seen and experienced in hospitals (but see section 7 below).

Although students *could* learn in the community about most of the illnesses, disease and disabilities in a core curriculum, there is a smaller proportion of conditions where learning *must* take place in the community because they are not found in hospitals. The specific community-based objectives learning about illnesses, disease, and disability will depend on the particular strategy each medical school adopts to cover its core curriculum. The range can be from almost the complete list of core conditions ot a selected subset.

One of the benefits of learning in general practice is the opportunity to see patients with *undifferentiated problems* where the symptoms have not been organized into syndromes or diagnoses. Observing and exploring the initial presentation of chest pain may be a more valuable learning experience for a student than meeting the same patient in a cardiology (or gastroenterology, or rheumatology) clinic. Students in general practice can learn about the diagnostic process from the start, and can also explore different problem-solving strategies as well as those that are common to primary and secondary care.

Learning about disease processes or pathology (GMC Objective 1 (c)) will probably be covered initially in an institutional setting, but in a fully integrated course students should also address such issues in primary care. They can learn about infection as they consider microbiological investigations or inflammation from the relevant blood tests in, for example, a patient with rheumatoid disease. Degeneration can be explored with X-rays of osteoarthritis, and concepts of neoplasia from cervical cytology.

The range of possible objectives in this field is great. Most examples are drawn from those topics which are best learned in the community, although some could equally well be addressed in hospitals.

Sample objectives

Students should be able to:-

- demonstrate a knowledge of the *range of problems* that are presented to doctors in primary care, and the *range of solutions* that have been developed for their recognition, investigation, prevention, and treatment;
- describe the clinical course of common infections, their appropriate investigations, and management;
- describe and defend a differential diagnosis for a patient presenting acutely with (e.g.) epigastric pain, backpain, headache, etc;
- demonstrate an understanding of the pathological processes underlying the common diseases of general practice;
- demonstrate a caring attitude towards people with disabilities.

6. LEARNING HOW TO ASSESS PATIENTS (GMC Objective 2(a))

In traditional medical education, basic skills of history-taking and physical examination have been learnt in the hospital setting, because that was where the clinical teachers worked, and where patients were perceived to be available for learning experience. Both these premises have become false, since there is now a substantial body of trained clinical tutors in general practice and patients in hospital are often there for very short times and are no longer available for learning. Students therefore need to learn clinical method from history-taking to assessing patients' problems and formulating plans in the community.

Communication skills are a particularly important aspect of clinical method that students need to learn. This is a field that postgraduate teachers in general practice have pioneered, and where many have become skilled exponents (see Pendleton *et al.* 1984; Tate 1994). Most undergraduate general practice courses now expect students to conduct consultations on their own, often with videorecording and feedback. The community can be an ideal setting for students to develop skills they have started to learn in a classroom setting. In particular, they should learn to make use of the context both in history-taking and in interpretation of the findings.

Students also need the opportunity to develop their skills in physical examination. They may have learnt the basic in skills laboratories or by experience with each other but continual practice is needed in a range of skills from examining limbs to auscultating chests and from using a sphygmomanometer to otoscopy.

Sample objectives

Objectives in this area will be closely allied to the general objectives of proficiency in basic clinical method and those to be achieved within other settings. Students may arrive with specific personal objectives especially in the field of physical examination and assessment, for example, to be able to:

- examine the back;
- use an otoscope and interpret the findings;
- assess a patient's mental state.

Other objectives, such as communication skills, may be particularly applicable in the one-to-one relationship of many community settings, for example, students should be able to:

- establish effective relationships with patients;
- use open and closed questions appropriately to elicit the history;
- use silence effectively;
- demonstrate empathy when appropriate;
- recognize non-verbal cues;
- adapt their information-giving to the patient's needs;
- use appropriate language.

7. LEARNING ABOUT THERAPY (GMC Objective 1(g))

There has been a tendency for concepts of therapy to be limited to pharmacology and therapeutics, often taught and examined as a separate subject, or to a knowledge of appropriate surgical procedures. Experience of medical students in general practice suggested they often had a poor grasp of the wider principles of management as applied to common diseases and problems (such as hypertension, asthma, or stroke). GMC objective (1(g)) is very detailed in specifying a knowledge of the principles of therapy. It includes the management of acute and chronic illness, disease and disability, drug and non-drug therapies and the relief of pain and care of the dying.

A community perspective which looks at the context of all these forms of therapy will broaden the objectives in this area. For instance, in considering the prescription and administration of drugs it will be important for students to learn about factors affecting patient compliance. There are also a whole range of objectives that relate to rehabilitation and community care.

The explicit inclusion of care of the dying is important here since it could be argued that effective palliative care involves the whole range of therapeutic resources. If students understand this, they will have a model on which to base all other therapeutic decisions. Palliative care requires a careful history to establish the nature of the patient's problems (physical, psychological, and social); as precise a diagnosis as possible for each symptom; and then a range of approaches. This range includes the best, most imaginative, choice of drugs, recognizing the interactions and side-effects of each. However, non-drug interventions (e.g. psychotherapy, counselling, physical therapies, and alternative therapies) and down-to-earth expert nursing are equally important in palliative care. Students need to appreciate and learn these different facets. Palliative care commonly takes place in community settings that include community hospitals (or GP hospitals) and hospices, as well as the many patients cared for at home. Good liaison with specialists, and with Macmillan Nurses exemplifies good practice in this area. However, even in the absence of formal palliative care, general practice is an ideal setting for students to learn the principles of therapy.

Sample objectives

Students should be able to:

- devise a suitable management plan for patients with common acute illnesses;
- devise a suitable management plan for patients with common chronic diseases (e.g. diabetes, asthma, hypertension, osteoarthritis, depression);
- demonstrate an understanding of the way drug actions contribute to drug interactions and side-effects;
- select appropriate non-drug treatments for patients with relevant problems;
- describe the roles of physiotherapists, occupational therapists, counsellors, psychologists, chiropodists, and other relevant therapists;
- devise a suitable management plan for a terminally ill patient.

8. LEARNING ABOUT MANAGEMENT AND PROVISION OF HEALTH CARE
(GMC Objective 1(l))

Management includes 'experience in administration and planning; appropriate use of resources, and appreciation of economic and practical constraints affecting health care; and willingness to participate in bodies which advise, plan, and assist the development and administration of medical services' (Fairhurst *et al.* 1995, quoting from the GMC's 1987 recommendations on training of specialists). While some of these objectives can reasonably be deferred to postgraduate training, as the GMC clearly implied at the time, there are fundamental management concepts which every medical graduate, however junior, needs to understand and apply. These include personal time management, goal-setting, prioritizing, delegation of tasks, the ability to work in groups (both for learning and for task-achievement), and the appreciation of the economic dimension.

There are also parallels between the clinical task of diagnosis and the management task of problem-solving which are themselves educational (Fairhurst *et al.* 1995). If students appreciate the constraints placed on diagnosis by having limited information, they will understand the importance of gathering sufficient information when addressing a problem of organization, staffing, or resourcing. Similarly, by appreciating the importance of good, open, sensitive, empathic communication in the clinical setting, their management skills will be enhanced by transferring this attitude to their work with colleagues.

Medical audit was introduced as an educational activity, but it also has a management function, which can often be integrated with the educational. It is far better that medical practitioners feel able to collaborate with health care managers in both the design and interpretation of audit, than that they perceive management audit as an external threat!

Many of these objectives are suitable for community settings. General practices are small organizations involved in the management and provision of health care. They work on a scale which it is easier for students to perceive both the problems and the solutions. At the same time, larger organizations such as Medical Audit Advisory Groups and Health Commissions with their Public Health Departments can provide broader perspectives.

Sample objectives

Students should be able to:

* demonstrate an understanding of the principles of management (planning, prioritizing, delegating, monitoring, evaluating);
* demonstrate effective personal time management;
* recognize the constraints and implications of finite resources in health care;
* plan and execute a simple audit of health care.

9. LEARNING ABOUT INFORMATION-PROCESSING (GMC Objective 2(c))

The amount of published medical knowledge is increasing exponentially. No individual can now expect to keep fully informed just by reading a number of journals regularly. This information explosion implies that future medical graduates will need a different range of skills in information-handling. In particular they will need the competence to handle electronic information retrieval systems. Computer-aided learning (CAL) is becoming a standard medium in medical education. Students need to be proficient in using this. Most students are now highly computer literate before starting medical school but, for others, training in basic skills is still needed and medical informatics, already part of some undergraduate curricula, will soon be universal.

In terms of accessing scientific data, general practice computing is not yet well developed compared with what students may be used to in their medical schools. This is likely to change over the next few years with access to networks. It will affect the retrieval and application of evidence within general practice and will provide opportunities for students to learn how to appraise the use of such evidence. On the other hand, computerized patient management systems are already much better developed in general practice. The community is an ideal setting for students to learn the values (and limitations) of electronic patient records, electronic linkages between hospitals, health commissions and general practitioners, and other applications. Students in community settings have the opportunity to learn the difficulties in recording contextual information and the sources of error in any recording.

The rapidly changing nature of computing in general practice also illustrates the importance for students of an enlightened attitude towards change (GMC Objective 3(j)). Familiarity with one computer system will be of limited value in using a different system, but the principles of computer systems in general practice are highly relevant to any medical graduate.

Sample objectives:

Students should be able to:

- use a personal computer for word-processing, spreadsheet, and simple statistical manipulations;
- show an appreciation of the principles of data protection, confidentiality, and security;
- use a clinical information system to record, and retrieve patient clinical data;
- access and use an electronic network to carry out a literature search on a community topic.

10. LEARNING ATTITUDES (GMC Objectives 3(a—l))

An 'attitude' is an abstract construct, with different meanings in different contexts. While it may have a precise meaning in certain psychological research settings, in educational terms it is used rather more generally, almost as a synonym for values. It refers to a predisposition to act in a certain way, to think one way or the other about a particular situation, to hold to certain given propositions. 'Respect . . . without prejudice' (GMC Objective 3(a)) implies that the student will not act in a different way towards people of different backgrounds, language, or culture. Since most medical students come from middle-class backgrounds, some may unconsciously have acquired a prejudiced view of people from other backgrounds: medical education must enable them to modify such an attitude and experience in communities should be a major factor in this.

Likewise, there is a risk that medical students, having been high achievers at school, and succeeding in a course that is certainly intellectually challenging, might hold the view that they, as part of the medical profession, are (almost) omniscient and omnipotent. This is not a helpful attitude, as it predisposes to arrogance, and leads to despair when the truth eventually dawns! Students should acquire awareness of their personal limitations, and of the need to seek help when necessary (GMC Objective 3(h)). This will include seeking help from other team members and requires the development of team-working skills and exploring attitudes to other health professionals. Awareness of the need for continuing professional development (GMC Objective 3(k)) should be developed throughout the course. The more personal one-to-one setting of general practice can help to cultivate these attitudes.

General practitioners are probably even more aware than specialist doctors of the need to cope with uncertainty (GMC Objective 3(d)). Very often a patient's symptoms cannot be fully explained, either at the first visit, or even after a period of time. Balancing the probability of serious pathology against the risks of harmful over-investigation is a dilemma common to general practitioners, which students can use to learn about the problem of uncertainty.

The word *care* appears within these objectives (GMC Objectives 3(e),(f)). Caring is primarily an attitude. When that attitude is present, then knowledge and skills are deployed, but without the attitude, the knowledge and skills remain unused. Caring is not the prerogative of any part of the health care professions but the motto of the Royal College of General Practitioners (*cum scientiae caritas*—knowledge with compassion) is a reminder that this ethos has been central to primary medical care.

Modelling is a powerful learning process, in which the learner identifies with the model. The stronger the identification the greater the learning. There is both a challenge and a warning here, especially if students have a close relationship with a tutor by virtue of the time spent with them. In community settings this can be all day for several weeks. The attitudes that govern tutors' actions (usually implicit, but sometimes quite explicit) will rub off on to the student. For this reason, tutors in general practice should give thought to their own attitudes, and when appropriate, make them explicit.

Sample objectives

This is an area where specific assessable objectives can be hard to define. However, it is possible to look at some areas where the community is particularly relevant. Some sample attitudinal objectives are found in previous sections. In addition the student should be able to:

- explore the degree of uncertainty in a first presentation of a condition and the methods that may be used to cope with it;
- define the moral and ethical implications of a management decision;
- exhibit curiosity and the ability to question the rationale for decisions;
- exhibit a willingness to discuss personal limitations and to seek help;
- show constructive approaches as a member of a group or team.

CONCLUSION

This chapter has described a number of objectives of undergraduate medical education that can be met in a community setting. It will be appreciated that many of these objectives are not unique to the community and can clearly also be achieved within hospitals or other institutions such as skills laboratories. This reinforces the importance of integration and of discussion with students about the best way to use time spent in the community.

Part Three
Approaches for learning

To follow a hospital-attending about the wards and see what he does in his daily routine may enable the student to pick up many practical points but it is not medical education. (James Ewing 1916)

Having considered the aims and objectives of a medical course and the broad outlines of a curriculum, it is now necessary to look at educational methods and how these can be used in community settings.

The first part of Part III, from Chapters 5 to 9, focuses on the different approaches that can be used: these range from large lecture theatres to one-to-one attachments. The advantages and disadvantages of each approach will be discussed. There will also be consideration of the extent to which they can be applied in the community. The second part, Chapters 10 to 15, then provides detailed applications of these approaches. Specific examples are given on how the approaches can be used to achieve various objectives within a community setting.

5 One-to-one teaching

A major difference of attachments in community settings is that students commonly have a one-to-one relationship with their tutors. In the traditional hospital setting specialists work with firms which often include several students. The consultant with a huge retinue gathering round a bedside is more redolent of a past period than of current practice but much clinical teaching still takes place in the setting of a firm. Even if students of today often have individual tutors for certain purposes, they are seldom attached to them as ever-watchful apprentices for long periods. General practitioners have usually found that they can only manage one student at a time in a consulting room or on a visiting round. This enables a much closer relationship to develop between tutor and pupil. During attachments to a GP tutor many learning opportunities are available. Many of these encompass the possibility of discussion and reflection on a one-to-one basis and these are the subject of this chapter.

THE STUDENT IN THE CONSULTING ROOM

Central to any attachment will be the opportunity to sit in the consulting room and be involved in encounters between doctors and patients. Sadly, this experience has often been misused in the past: the picture of the bored student suffering from the 'wallpaper syndrome', stuck in a corner as patients appear to enter and depart with devastating speed, trying to gather a few crumbs of learning.

The consultation, however, should be a highly valued learning experience. Spence did say that everything else in medicine derives from the consultation. Even if that were an overstatement, the meeting between doctor and patient is still an essential element of learning.

It is important for the student to appreciate at the start of an attachment that sitting in on surgery consultations is fundamentally different from many types of clinical experience in hospitals. Students need to understand that:

- The general practice consultation is private, sometimes intimate, often building on a relationship which has been developed over many years. For this reason, patients may ask to be seen without a student more frequently than in hospital settings.

- Consultations often contain sensitive information about psychological and social aspects of patients' lives.
- They are privileged observers of the interaction between doctor and patient, and that confidentiality is of the greatest importance.

As the consultation is primarily for the benefit of the patient the tutor may need to make certain ground rules clear. Students need to understand that they should dress and conduct themselves in a way that disrupts the consultation as little as possible. It is also necessary to state whether and when the student is welcome to interrupt dialogue between the doctor and the patient.

Setting the scene

Students sometimes react with bewilderment at the process of general practice consultations. Compared to the defined framework of, for example, a gynaecology clinic, general practice surgeries not only contain a kaleidoscope of different problems, but also present a much wider range of types of approach. In most hospital medical clinics, the nature of the problem has usually been fairly well defined, and the role of the doctor clear-cut (e.g. make a diagnosis, advise on management). This is not the case in general practice consultations where:

- Consultations are rapid.
- The presenting symptom may not even be the reason for consultation.
- Patients consult for problems which are ill defined, and often undefinable.
- Patient problems cross the boundaries of conventional medical problems.
- The GP makes use of his knowledge of probability and of the natural history of common conditions to manage large elements of uncertainty.
- The GP uses past knowledge of the patient as a key input to defining the problem and making management decisions.

There is a real danger that, when students first arrive in general practice, they see an impossibly confusing range of problems. They may perceive the doctor as making a series of apparently irrational decisions at very high speed. The tutor needs to be explicit about some of the processes used during the first few surgery sessions.

The tutor also needs to be alert to management approaches which have become second nature to a doctor in general practice, and have a safe and sound basis, which may appear illogical or dangerous to the student. Thus, for example, if the student believes that 20% of patients presenting with headache may have a brain tumour, then a management approach which concentrates on psychosocial history may appear dangerously negligent. Achievement of objectives concerning understanding disease and assessment from a community perspective may be hampered if the scene is not set properly. Students must be introduced to the differences between community and hospital medicine if they are to make the best use of the opportunities.

A structured approach helps students become oriented in an initially unfamiliar clinical environment. One approach to providing a framework for such a discussion is for students to keep a log book. Log books can be valuable in helping students to analyse what has occurred in a surgery. They can also be used to collect information relating to specific course objectives, or as means of remembering points which the student wishes to follow up later, either on his or her own or with the tutor.

When analysing a surgery consultation, the tutor should be explicit about the varying roles which the GP takes from time to time, sometimes within the same consultation. This could, for example, be framed in terms of Stott and Davis' (1979) model of the potential for each consultation (see Box 1). This model can help students appreciate the variety of activity taking place in a simple consultation, and thus learn more about the breadth of an individual patient's health needs.

An important framework for students is to learn to consider each consultation in terms of a biopsychosocial model. They should be asked to note the relative contribution of:

- The biological illness with which the patient presents.
- Psychological factors, fears, feelings, and expectations that affect presentation or management.
- Social and structural factors affecting presentation or management.

This is the so-called triple (or triaxial) diagnosis in clinical, individual, and contextual terms. A typical example, familiar to undergraduates, would be the medical student who presented with tonsillitis and cervical lymphadenopathy (the clinical diagnosis) but who was anxious because of having seen a patient with Hodgkin's lymphoma (the individual diagnosis). The proximity of examinations may be part of a contextual diagnosis that also affects process and outcome.

How to structure the surgery time

Students need time to ask questions, reflect, and learn from the experience. Additional time has to be set aside when medical students are part of surgery sessions. Two methods of discussing patients are in common use. The first is to discuss each patient briefly with the student before the next one is seen. The second is to save the discussion until the end of surgery. It is much more difficult to engage a student's interest without regular interaction: in general, leaving all discussion until the end of surgery will produce a bored student. However, if discussions between seeing patients are not going to disrupt an appointment system, time has to be set aside. It is probably reasonable to build in an extra two minutes per patient when a student is present to allow for brief discussion of individual patients. This may also be accomplished by building gaps into the surgery so that, for example, every fifth patient is followed by a space if consultations are booked at ten minute intervals and every fourth patient is followed by a space if consultations are booked at seven and a half minute intervals. If surgeries are normally booked

---

Box 1   The exceptional potential of the general practice consultation (from Stott and Davis 1979)

Management of the presenting problem	Management of continuing problems
Modification of help-seeking behaviour	Opportunistic health promotion

at five minute intervals, then there is a question whether this provides an adequate educational environment. The danger of the 'wallpaper syndrome' has already been mentioned. Students do not enjoy being 'wallpaper', and they do not learn unless they are engaged by the tutor. If there are times when, perhaps through pressure of time, a tutor needs to see patients in rapid succession without much reference to the student, then this should be made clear to the student, with an opportunity being offered later to ask questions.

Even two minutes between consultations is hardly leisurely, and it is important to be explicit to students that no attempt will be made to cover all the issues which arise for an individual patient. Both tutor and student need to be selective about what is to be addressed, and agree that topics which require longer discussion can be dealt with at the end of surgery or even on a later occasion. This is easier if there has been prior agreement on some main objectives for a session.

Involving students in taking histories

An important aspect of learning about people and their disease is for students to have the opportunity to talk to patients themselves. Students are used to spending an appreciable part of their time on hospital wards and in clinics taking histories from patients. Although arranging this may be more difficult in general practice, it should be a priority for the tutor both to maintain student interest and to encourage them to take a broader perspective when talking with patients.

There are several ways of involving students in talking to patients in the course of routine surgery sessions. These include:

- to ask the student to take part of the history during the course of a consultation which the GP is carrying out;
- to identify, shortly after the start, that a consultation would be suitable for the student to carry out and then arrange for the student to take a history and/or examine the patient in a separate consulting room;
- to book patients specifically to see the student before they see the GP.

Involving the student during the GP's own history taking can start with prompts such as: 'What else would you like to know about Mrs Acton's problem?' or 'Would you like to ask some further questions about Mr Barking's cough?' Such questions are usually fairly easy to introduce without making the patient feel uncomfortable. However, this technique may induce a sense of permanent anxiety in some students who will then sit in fear of being asked to take over the consultation. There is a fine line between producing a state of wakeful anticipation and one of unremitting nervousness in the student. Use of this technique therefore needs discussion and agreement with the student.

Often, it will become apparent very early in a consultation that it would be appropriate for the student to take the history. If an additional room is available, then the patient can be asked whether he or she has time to see the student first and the doctor afterwards. Although somewhat artificial for the patient, this technique can allow the doctor to orient the student as to the line of questioning which should be adopted and fill in with some background knowledge of the patient. Whether or not a separate room is available, the tutor may choose to use the opportunity to observe the student taking a history. With some patients it will be quite acceptable for the doctor and student to change chairs and for the student to take the history with the doctor as observer.

A third approach is for patients to see a student first. This is the preferred method of giving students contact with patients in the consulting room, and should be arranged for all students at some time during their time in general practice. One way to approach this is to book some patients specifically to see the student. Many surgeries inform patients that a student will be present when the appointment is made. The additional step required for a student consultation is for the receptionist to say to specified patients in a surgery (e.g. one near the start and one at the end)—'Dr Canning has a student with him today. Can I book you to see the student doctor first, and you would then see Dr Canning afterwards?' The receptionist then books separate appointments for the patient with the student and, 15 to 20 minutes later, for the GP. Booking separate consultations generally requires access to a separate room. Student consultations may save the GP time since, while a student is seeing a patient on his or her own, the GP may be able to see several other patients on his surgery list. If no separate room is available for the student consultations then patients may be booked for the student either before the normal surgery start time, or as the last patient of the surgery. Either of these approaches enables the tutor to be doing something else, (e.g. signing letters or prescriptions), while the student is consulting.

Whichever approach is taken, the patients themselves may often be regarded as 'tutors' as they will often help the student through the process.

Several criteria need to be met for effective learning to occur in this way:

- a suitable comfortable and private setting;
- a willing, consenting patient;
- assured confidentiality;
- adequate listening skills;
- a relevant framework for the interview, which might be generated during it.

Involving students in physical examination

It is on the whole easier to involve the student in physical examinations than in taking a history. It will often be natural for the student to be asked to repeat an examination which has just been carried out by the tutor. However, even this simple procedure requires some thought.

Any examination needs the consent of the patient. The tutor *must* always ask if the student may examine an individual. The tutor also needs to be aware of situations where it might be difficult for a patient to express unease or to withhold consent. For instance it may be better to seek consent before a patient is already partially undressed or lying flat; it may also be better to speak to the patient in the privacy of an examination room before the student enters. In these situations, the doctor's role as advocate for the patient must take precedence over the role as tutor.

The time which the student takes to do the physical examination should not be taken as the opportunity for the tutor to write up his or her notes. Students need to be observed while carrying out physical examinations so that faulty or clumsy techniques can be rectified. Students should also be given the opportunity to examine a range of normal as well as abnormal signs. If students are only invited to examine when the doctor has found an abnormality that will be a powerful clue. They may agree they can pick up an abnormal sign rather than appear foolish and unskilled. Students need to feel secure that they can say an examination appears normal. Of course, the history is also a powerful sensitizer to picking up physical signs in all doctors. One is more likely to hear a rhonchus in a patient who is known to have asthma. Students' expectations when examining patients have to be considered. The anecdote is told of a cardiologist who was teaching students about heart signs in mitral stenosis. The sounds they were expected to hear were beautifully described and illustrated. Each student in turn used the stethoscope the cardiologist offered and after examining the patient said how they had heard the opening snap and the murmur clearly. The cardiologist then unscrewed the head of the stethoscope and took out the wad of cotton wool placed there earlier. Such an approach is unkind and humiliating, and not to be recommended, but it is a reminder that expectations are very powerful and learning effective clinical skills requires a reduction of extraneous cues.

Students should use opportunities in the surgery to develop and improve their clinical examination skills with the benefit of a one-to-one tutor. Increasingly, learning the basic clinical examination skills will be a specified part of education in the community. Experiments have already shown the opportunities for a significant proportion of such teaching to be delivered outside traditional hospital sessions (see the chapters by Collerton and Booton, and Oswald in Part IV). Casual examination of patients during routine surgery may not be sufficient for more systematic teaching of this nature. It may be necessary to organize some patients to return for specific sessions where additional time is set aside for learning these skills. Such additional time and resources may be uneconomic for individual students and this approach may be better for a small group of students.

Involving students in management decisions

In the past, opportunity to be involved in the formulation of management plans has played a comparatively small part of student experience in hospital, although curricular development is changing this. However, it has always been a central part of almost every general practice consultation and students can be involved in the process. Shared formulation of management plans helps the student to understand the role of the GP in practising safe medicine while understanding the importance of diagnostic probabilities, and being able to live with uncertainty. Involving students in the negotiation of management decisions with patients is valuable for them as they learn a patient-centred approach to management.

It is often easy to involve a student at the stage in a consultation where a management decision is being made. The tutor may, for example, turn to the student and say: 'How would you explain this problem to Mr Deane?', or 'What would you advise Mr Ealing to do about this problem?' When students are asked to take a history themselves, they should be specifically told to think about how they would manage the problem and to formulate this in terms of the three aspects of management that mirror the triple diagnosis in clinical, individual, and contextual terms mentioned on p. 57.

Although this approach is important to enable students to develop competence in problem-solving it has to be managed with care. Consideration has to be given to the feelings of both patients and students. Patients should not be made unduly anxious by student suggestions. Equally, students should not feel that their proposals have been considered rubbish by doctor or patient. If the plan is to be presented in front of the patient, the tutor needs a strategy to deal with an unacceptable approach without confusing the patient or humiliating the student. If a potentially faulty management plan is to be discussed, then it may helpful to generalize the problem beyond that of the individual patient, and for the tutor to explain to the patient what is being done.

Sometimes, students will lack sufficient knowledge to formulate a management plan, and it is important not to demoralize them by continually asking questions to which they are unable to respond. In other circumstances, the tutor may know that the proposed management is unlikely to find favour with the patient. With care, the student's approach can be developed interactively between the student, patient, and tutor.

VISITING PATIENTS AT HOME

A major opportunity offered by community based attachments is the ability to visit patients at home. Home visits offer unparalleled opportunities to explore objectives which relate to the presentation and management of illness, environmental and social determinants of disease, and human relationships. Tutors should therefore ensure that home visits play a regular part in the experiences arranged for a student.

Often, home visits will involve accompanying the GP or another member of the primary care team in the course of their normal visits. In these circumstances, the opportunities to involve students in taking histories, examining patients, and formulating management plans are similar to those described in the previous section. However, there should also be opportunities for students to carry out independent visits to patients at home. Such visits are often regarded by students as the most valuable and enjoyable part of their time in the community, although they are sometimes nervous about visiting patients on their own at home. However, although it is a privilege rather than a right for them to enter patients' homes, it is extremely uncommon for them not to be made welcome.

There are four main opportunities for involving students in independent home visits.

1. Follow-up of acute visits in general practice

There are many situations where a doctor undertakes an acute visit, and where it may be valuable for the student to follow-up the patient even though the doctor had not planned a revisit. For example, if an elderly patient is seen at home with acute on chronic bronchitis, the doctor's normal follow-up might well be to tell the patient to call again if the infection had not resolved within a few days. There would not necessarily be any medical need for a revisit but an arrangement might be made for the student to visit the patient again in, say, three days. This gives the student the opportunity to learn about the natural history of acute illnesses, as well as exploring other aspects of the patient's situation.

2.Visiting patients with acute problems: initial assessment

More experienced students may gain valuable experience in assessing illness and formulating management plans by visiting acutely ill patients at home on their own. The simplest way of arranging this is for the tutor in a general practice to keep an eye on the visit book during the course of a morning surgery. If a visit request looks suitable for a student to carry out independently and is in easy reach, the tutor can then phone the patient or carer to ask if the student may visit first. During this phone call a few apposite questions can determine the suitability of the situation for an independent visit and the tutor can reassure the patient that this is not in place of the doctor's visit. The student will then make the visit and will return to report back and discuss the assessment and the proposed management. Later, during the routine visiting round, tutor and student will visit together; the assessment can be confirmed and the plan negotiated with the patient. While the opportunity for this sort of visit may not present very frequently, it can be a valuable learning experience for students, and usually receives very positive feedback from students.

3. Patients with long-term medical problems: visits in the community

Long-term medical problems provide many opportunities for students to achieve important learning objectives related to patients' reactions to illness and disability and the care and rehabilitation of the chronically ill and the disabled. A proper understanding of many of these issues requires that students spend considerable time with the patients themselves. As the proportion of community-based medical education increases students will need to have more of this patient contact within the community setting.

Visiting patients with chronic illness or disability in their own homes is an ideal method of providing experience of these issues. Such visits often give students time to explore properly the many facets of care. They can see at first hand how patients manage and what resources, aids, and adaptations are required. Patients within their own home will be more relaxed and in control. This enables them to feel free about explaining their situation to students, including their views on the services they receive. In this situation, the patients take on the role of tutors in a one-to-one situation.

Organization of such experience is helped if practices maintain a bank of patients who are suitable for this sort of independent visit and have agreed to see students regularly. Most practices could probably identify several patients who would be willing to be visited by a student, say six times a year. Identification in advance avoids the need for a doctor to telephone and ask patients to see a student at the last minute, although it may be necessary to confirm nearer the time that the patient is still able and willing to participate.

Independent visits for this purpose should take time. These are not ten minute interviews. At least one hour should be available if students are to gain the best benefit from the experience. Patients and students need to be aware of this, especially when an appointment is being negotiated. Many an independent visit has failed because the student arrives to find that the patient is being taken out in 15 minutes or because someone else calls. Student travelling arrangements must be considered. Students do not always have their own transport. A willing and interesting patient may live a long distance from easily accessible public transport. Sometimes community staff need to be willing to arrange to take and collect the student. Finally, people are rightly concerned about strangers entering their homes. Students should have suitable identification. This should include a letter of introduction from the doctor and a student union card with a picture.

4. Patients with long-term medical problems: hospital discharge planning

It is not only community tutors who might wish to organize student visits to patients at home. Some medical schools are starting to use discharge planning as a specific focus of undergraduate teaching. Discharge planning is particularly important for the elderly and other patients with long term medical problems, where careful discharge arrangements may be crucial for the successful rehabilitation of the patient at home. Learning from such planning is best achieved when students are involved on both sides of the interface. Prior to discharge, the student needs to be able to identify steps which have been taken to enable the patient to cope effectively when back in the community. After discharge, the student can carry out an independent visit to see whether the arrangements have actually been adequate, whether the pre-discharge judgements of the patient's abilities have proved to be well founded in the home situation, and whether the planned community resources are actually available and able to deliver what was expected of them. Visits of this nature will generally be arranged from the hospital, although the students may wish to talk to members of the primary care team caring for the patient at home. They can be of considerable value to students, but they are relatively difficult to organize. It is important that there is follow-up after the home visits to enable students to reflect on what they have learnt in the experience. This can be effectively carried out in a seminar where several students have had the opportunity to follow-up patients after discharge. Both hospital and community tutors can usefully contribute to such seminars.

EXPERIENCE WITH OTHER MEMBERS OF THE PRIMARY HEALTH CARE TEAM

So far, this chapter has considered the role of doctors and of patients in one-to-one education in the community. A third group of people can also be effectively involved. Most medical school curricula have been oriented around medical models of illness;

they have therefore concentrated on doctors' roles in caring for patients. The values which students acquire in medical schools have principally been those of other doctors. The community setting offers substantial opportunities for students to look at other models of care, and to learn about the roles of other team members in providing care for patients. Many objectives might be addressed by sessions with other staff members, such as:

- learning to communicate with other health professionals;
- learning about the relative roles of different members of the primary care team in the management of patients;
- developing attitudes which value other team members as health professionals in their own right.

Experience with other team members needs to be arranged with care. It is not sufficient for the student simply to be told that one afternoon will be spent with, for example, the health visitor. Without some preparation, such sessions can seem pointless to the student and reinforce negative attitudes. The tutor responsible for the student's programme should discuss with students how such sessions might relate to their own learning objectives. It is preferable if the discussion on objectives precedes the planning of the sessions so that it is clear why they are occurring at a particular time, although this may not be always logistically possible. It is also important for the tutor to ensure that the other team member is aware of the learning objectives of the course and the individual student. It may be worth providing a short briefing paper on attachments which should include a reminder to ask for the student's view on areas to be covered.

Although time with community nurses, health visitors, practice nurses, and reception staff are the commonest experiences arranged for students with members of the primary care team, there are many other people that students can learn from in the community setting. These include a diverse range such as midwife, social worker, alternative practitioner, physiotherapist, relaxation therapist, pharmacist, or counsellor. Individual experiences will depend on what services are available in individual practices and areas. The organization of such attachments in one medical school is discussed in Chapter 23. Students may need some direction in order to consider the activities of the more out of the ordinary workers, as part of their learning objectives. However, these atypical opportunities can help to promote attitudes of curiosity. Where a problem-based approach is being used, students should already be divergent in their thinking. They might wish to explore the availability of different workers, and the contribution they can make. Over time, it will be helpful if practices have a list of suitable contacts, and of people who are willing to have a brief discussion with students. A practice may have a good relationship with a local pharmacist who would be prepared to let students visit behind the scenes, or they may be aware of local osteopaths or acupuncturists who would be very pleased to discuss their approach.

Often it will be easier for students to discuss the role of other professionals if the discussion is related to a particular patient they have seen. When case reviews are taking place it may be appropriate to ask if a student can attend, although there may be problems with rules of confidentiality.

Social Services Departments and Care Managers have roles which it is particularly important for students to learn about. Unfortunately, many such departments are heavily overworked and find it difficult to give time to see students.

With all these practitioners, who may be more remote from the practice, it is important that some briefing is provided so that they use their time with students appropriately.

An attachment session

A typical attachment session should consist of:

- A *preparation period*. During this students will decide what questions they need to ask.
- An *observation period*. Students need the opportunity to see exactly what people are doing. Watching how staff members relate to patients and seeing their skills at first hand is more effective than description.
- A *discussion period*. Staff should ensure that they have time after the observation to discuss what the students saw, their feelings and their questions. This may be carried out by the tutor as well, but the students will learn more from the staff member.

Most members of the primary care team will welcome the opportunity to have occasional medical students with them. The request often results in a reciprocal one for the doctor to offer some time to a health visiting or nursing student. How experiences with individual team members might operate is discussed in later chapters.

CONCLUSION

This chapter has looked at the way that students can learn from one-to-one contacts with a variety of health professionals, patients, and doctors. One-to-one contact can be very time-consuming and it can also be very boring if the student is marginalized while professionals get on with their own work. It is therefore very important that tutors ask themselves various questions:

- Which objectives are best achieved in a one-to-one contact?
- Have the objectives for a session been clearly defined?
- Has sufficient time been set aside for discussion and reflection on the experience?

6 Learning on one's own: projects and independent tasks

In a learner-centred approach students identify their specific learning needs and seek to address them. They are encouraged to seek out and use the resources they need themselves. Many of these resources will be in libraries or, increasingly, accessed through computer networks. Students may also need to contact human resources, experts in a field or a sample of people who can be interviewed or complete questionnaires. Independent learning of this nature can extend from a brief task requiring a few hours to an extended project over several weeks. Developments in curricula and in educational method mean that students are more commonly engaged in this approach to learning. A core plus options curriculum means that several special study periods are set apart in which students will often carry out projects independently. The cardinal feature of problem-based learning is that, for a particular subject, a student, or group of students, identifies specific tasks that need to be carried out prior to feedback at the next seminar.

Independent learning will cover all settings including the community. Tutors in the community, including general practitioners, therefore have a role to play which may include suggesting suitable projects, identification of resources or supervision, and support.

SHORT OR LONG TASKS

When a problem-based learning approach is being used students will come to a surgery with several brief tasks that they need to perform between the initial and the feedback seminars (see Chapter 7). Some of these tasks can probably be addressed during the course of normal surgery work (e.g. How often do GPs prescribe antibiotics for respiratory infections?). Others tasks will require access to practice-based information (e.g. How does the practice ensure that a high proportion of eligible women have cervical smears carried out?). For some tasks, students may need to look at other community settings (e.g. What services are available in the community for drying-out alcoholics?). Tutors will be better prepared to help students with identifying the appropriate resources if they are aware of concurrent seminar work. They will be able to predict those tasks which students commonly bring and even prepare resource packs for them.

The other requirement is for more formal project work. There is no clear definition of a project which may last from one day to three months (or even longer if it is in an intercalated year). In any attachment of reasonable length the use of a project enables students to cover one issue in depth, and then to apply the findings from that experience to other similar issues. A special study module can allow an even greater depth of learning. In some medical schools, project work has been carried out for many years, and produced high quality work in the community, sometimes resulting in publication. The subject of the project may arise from the seminar work. Students will frequently have a broad idea of an area they wish to explore but the definition of a feasible project arises from discussion between student and tutor. The tutor may need to guide the student to refine the question they are asking. Students often come with very broad questions such as 'How well is asthma managed in general practice?' They need to consider which facets of such a question might be achievable within the time available and which approach they want to take. Approaches may range from a literature review to a small audit of a particular aspect in one practice. Often, the area of a student's interest may coincide with the interests of the practice, particularly those relating to audit. When this happens the student might be prepared to make small modification in what they want to do in order to work with others on an audit. However, students should never be pressured into doing a particular project simply because it is something that the practice needs to do. They should feel that they 'own' the project. Consequently, some audit projects may not be feasible, as there will not be time to complete the cycle unless there is an extended contact with the practice environment. On the other hand, it is possible to do projects that survey an aspect of care or that enable students to investigate the resources that are available.

RESOURCING A PROJECT

Students carrying out independent learning in a community setting need a number of resources. A shift of curricular time from core teaching to special study modules and more project work implies a shift of resources to meet the needs of a changing curriculum. There may be an increased need for staff time: students may need help in accessing records or learning how to use the computer system to do searches. Even if students can be expected to retrieve and replace files themselves, they need to learn about the filing system and they will need time to discuss issues of confidentiality. Sometimes, students return to their home area and ask to do a project within their local practice. Here, issues such as confidentiality need special care.

There will be need for protected time with the tutor to discuss the progress of the project and problems that are arising, and to reflect on any findings. It is sometimes easy to forget a student who is beavering away in a corner of the office, especially if clinical work is busy. However, students need opportunities for feedback throughout the project, not just when they are collecting results.

Other resources may be required. Where will the student work? Who will be responsible for typing and duplicating questionnaires? If a postal contact is part of the project who is responsible for the postal costs? All these are important aspects of planning project work.

SAMPLE PROJECTS

Examples of projects follow. First there are several 'mini-projects' suitable for two or three half-day sessions.

Evaluating diabetic care

Using a disease register or computer to get a list, extract the notes of a sample of patients with diabetes, and determine whether routine screening tests (as defined in a practice or district protocol) have been carried out at appropriate intervals.

Evaluating hypertensive care

Use requests for repeat prescriptions to provide a list of patients being treated for hypertension. Extract the notes of a sample of such patients and determine how frequently their blood pressure has been checked and whether control is satisfactory.

Assessing doctor—patient communication—1

Interview patients before and after consultations with the doctor. Determine whether they had asked all they wanted to ask, and if not, what had prevented them. At the most basic level, this could be done impromptu for two hours following on discussion between the tutor and student about the importance of addressing patients' concerns. An alternative would be to use a brief questionnaire given to a larger number of patients.

Assessing doctor—patient communication—2

Do patients understand what doctors say to them? Patients are interviewed after a consultation which the student has observed. Patients should be asked in advance whether they would be willing to see the student to answer a few questions after the consultation. The student's role would be to determine whether the patient understood what the doctor had said and to draw up a comparison between their perception of the information and the patient's. At a very basic level, this could again be done with little advanced planning, for one surgery session following a discussion between the tutor and student about the importance of good explanations.

The possibilities for a larger project are vast. The projects mentioned above could be extended.

Evaluating the care of a chronic illness

A longer project on diabetes and hypertension could include searching the literature in order to find criteria for evaluation (e.g. the appropriate routine tests or levels for control). It could also include discovering whether patients who appeared to have escaped follow-up had in fact done so, and if so why.

Evaluating doctor-patient communication

A project which involved designing a questionnaire for a semi-structured interview, and then interviewing patients in several practices in order to obtain generalizable results would be suitable as a project which could last for several weeks. Such an interview could consider aspects such as the time available, ability to complete their agenda, understanding of what the doctor said was wrong with them and understanding of the proposed management. This project might include a review of the literature on patient satisfaction.

Investigating the drinking or drug habits of a population

Some students are interested by problems that affect their own peer group. A population-based community project can enable them to investigate these safely. A student could use a practice list to derive a sample of people (e.g. people aged between 15 and 25) and then devise and distribute a questionnaire on aspects of lifestyle such as experence of alcohol or drug intake. Such a project can also help to develop understanding of epidemiology and environmental and social determinants of disease. At the same time they will learn about exploring existing evidence and contributing to the advancement of medical knowledge.

The individual case-study

Projects can also be based on an individual case-study. An in-depth analysis of individual cases can be used to fulfil several learning objectives. Students can be asked to consider the evidence for clinical interventions from a whole range of approaches. They can look at simple evidence of the accuracy of a particular test or the comparative effectiveness of a specific treatment. Alternatively, they could be asked to analyse critically a range of managements from both scientific and ethical viewpoints. The possibilities for this approach are as endless as the range of conditions seen in any general practice consultation session. The case-centred approach to problem-based learning can, of course, use similar methods but there are particular advantages of immediacy in working from a case seen by the students themselves, and directing them towards some of the public health, epidemiological, and ethical aspects.

7 Learning in small groups

Experience in clinical settings in the community, with its one-to-one and independent learning formats, needs to be supported by some more formal approaches to education. The principal formal method used in community-based medical education has been small-group work. For some time, small-group work has been widely used as an educational method within the discipline of general practice and most general practitioner tutors will be familiar and comfortable with it. As recognition is given to the importance of adult learning methods, so small-group techniques are increasingly gaining acceptance throughout the undergraduate course.

Group work may take place in medical school, hospital, or community premises. In many schools, general practices or health centres are being asked to accommodate small-group teaching if they have suitable sized rooms. Community-based tutors can be involved in any setting and may have three opportunities to participate.

First, there may be seminars which relate to the specific community aspects of the curriculum. During a community attachment the students may come together for sessions in which to share their individual experiences. There may also be specific seminars connected with particular objectives such as learning communication skills. In these instances the tutors will normally have a specific knowledge and expertise to share.

Second, in integrated courses, community-based personnel may be asked to function as group tutors. In such cases, such as problem-based learning groups, the material for discussion in the group may be related to a number of disciplines in which the tutors do not have personal expertise. They are being asked to provide educational expertise as group leaders. They are there to facilitate the learning process rather than to provide an expert resource. General practitioners, and others with long experience of group-learning methods, may have particular strengths as group facilitators.

Third, there may be involvement in interprofessional education. Even more challenging than producing an integrated curriculum is to provide education jointly with students of other professional groups such as nurses or social workers. Many of the problems which doctors have in working effectively in teams stem from a lack of understanding of the perspective of, or respect for the disciplines with whom they find themselves working. Effective collaboration between professional groups will be enhanced if links have been established from an early stage, including students' experience during their undergraduate training. Learning together with other professions in small groups can promote this. In this instance, tutors from different professions may well be working together. The final part of this chapter looks specifically at this area of learning which is likely to increase in coming years.

OBJECTIVES OF GROUP WORK

Compared to traditional methods of teaching like lectures, small groups are relatively expensive in tutor time. It is therefore important to be clear about the educational aims for which small groups are particularly effective. The aims of using small groups for learning can be considered under the headings of the three domains of learning: knowledge, skill, and attitudes. These can be summarized as follows:

1. Development of knowledge

- to encourage understanding in addition to imparting information;
- to improve integration and retention of factual knowledge.

2. Development of skills

- to develop problem-solving skills;
- to identify and practice particular skills (e.g. communication skills);
- to develop skills in oral presentation;
- to develop skills at working in teams.

3. Development of attitudes

- to enable students to take responsibility for their own learning;
- to identify their own learning needs and to develop strategies to meet those needs;
- to increase interest and motivation among students;
- to encourage collaboration rather than competition among students;
- to enhance students' self-esteem;
- to develop and broaden ethical awareness.

As well as development in cognitive, psychomotor, and affective domains, small groups provide an opportunity for assessment of learning, such as:

- to provide feedback to both students and tutors about the effectiveness of learning;
- to provide a forum where students may identify and address problems within their course;
- to enable feedback on the group process itself.

VARIETIES OF SMALL GROUPS

The term 'small group' defines only one parameter of this educational method, that is, group size. Small-group approaches can be developed in many ways to promote effective learning. Among these the following may be considered, although a particular group setting will involve a range of different tactics.

Task-oriented or process-oriented groups

In a task-oriented group the focus is on a specific area of knowledge or a particular skill that is to be obtained. Thus, a small group might concentrate on a problem about cerebrovascular accidents in order to develop factual understanding, or it might be devoted to acquiring skills in giving bad news.

The process-oriented group is concerned about its own development and learning process. It will consider the way that the group members tackle and develop a problem, looking at issues such as motivation and collaboration. There will be a particular emphasis on interpersonal skills and on attitudes.

In reality, most educational groups will be concerned with particular tasks but it is important that some time (whether an individual session or part of a session) is used to examine the process. This enables important attitudinal objectives to be picked up and evolved.

Problem-based or topic-based groups

Groups may be used effectively for learning about well-defined topics. Thus, the epidemiology of primary care might be the subject of a group where students share their experience of patients they have seen during an attachment in general practice. Topics such as dealing with difficult patients are suitable for a group communication-skills session. However, there is a danger with single topic sessions that they can become a vehicle for a mini-lecture from the tutor. An alternative approach is to base the session on a particular problem, which can range from a paper problem to a real case. This is the basis of problem-based learning (discussed in Chapter 2). There is increasing interest in the use of small groups in medical schools as a vehicle for this approach (see Bligh 1995).

Tutor-centred or learner-centred groups

In some small groups, the tutor takes an active role in leading the group discussion. This is more than simply presenting the starter material. The tutor continues to direct the flow of the discussion, preventing it from moving into areas the tutor sees as irrelevant. There is often a question-and-answer approach between tutor and students, and discussion is often directed through the tutor. Classically, in a tutor-centred group, the tutor is at a focal point (for instance next to a flipchart or whiteboard) and will often be the main contributor.

In learner-centred groups, the role of the tutor is less prominent: indeed the tutor can even leave the group for part of the time, enabling the students to continue the work of the group on their own. The role of the tutor is to listen carefully, to note problems that the group is encountering, and to consider ways in which the group's learning can be developed. These may include:

- Answering questions raised by the group. This may not always be by direct answers. At times, the tutor will reflect the question in such a way as to move the group on to a different way of thinking.
- Providing information about suitable learning resources, when requested by the group.
- Occasional interjections to challenge the group to consider alternative approaches that might be helpful.

In a learner-centred group the tutor appears solely as part of the group, or may even be positioned outside the group (as long as they can hear and see the group interaction). The tutor will also not be a main contributor in terms of time spent talking.

Tutors can find working with learner-centred groups quite threatening. There is less control of the group. This produces real fears that the group will fail to achieve important learning objectives. Another fear is that discussion will stray into areas beyond the competence of the tutor. Tutors need to realize that their aim is not to be an expert resource for all learning needs. The tutor works in two ways: they encourage students to think through issues clearly, and they are there to direct students where to find the necessary information or resource when requested.

Internally resourced or externally resourced groups

In an *externally resourced* group, an expert, who may have different expertise than the group leader, comes to provide the facts or skills that the students need to learn. Factual areas might include information about the organization of the health service, the roles of a team member, the diagnosis of skin complaints, or the management of the terminally ill. Skill areas might be cardiopulmonary resuscitation or a specific examination technique. This is a model widely used in vocational training for general practice. The expert does not have to provide a mini-lecture to the group. The group may decide itself what areas it wishes the external resource person to discuss. This can be done in advance and sent to the expert, it can be done at the beginning of the session, or it can be done interactively throughout the session. An important source of external resources are patients or carers who have to deal with a specific condition.

The danger with externally resourced groups is that the experts (whether patient or professional) dominate the discussion and do not relate their input to the objectives of the session or the students' learning needs. Briefing of experts is therefore essential.

Where the students themselves have to find out the answers to problems which they identify, the group is described as *internally resourced*. This is the conventional approach in problem-based learning. A concern of many tutors is that internally resourced groups will miss out on large areas of important facts or will misinterpret the information and the evidence that they get. Often, this will be remedied by other students who have considered the same areas and who challenge the presenter. If this fails to happen then it is possible for the tutor to challenge gently the findings and suggest that the evidence needs to be reconsidered. In an integrated curriculum, where group tutors do not have expertise in all the areas being considered, this concern may be even stronger. However, when information is presented, it is often apparent if some confusion has arisen. Tutors become adept at picking up areas that are questionable and prompting the group to explore further. (For general practitioners this is very similar to picking up cues in a consultation.) If doubt remains, the tutor can always contact an expert themselves. As the aim of small-group work is to develop critical powers in students, whatever happens, the situation is better than one where students listen to, and misinterpret, lectures, or where a lecturer provides personal, but unproven, impressions rather than information based on evidence.

FACILITATING A SMALL GROUP

Depending on the nature of the curriculum of an individual medical school, students will have a range of experience of group work from minimal to extensive. The tutor who is meeting a group for the first time needs to establish their level of experience, discuss the aims of the group, and agree the method of working. Some students approach seminars in the expectation of being the passive recipients of information. If they are being provided with a tutor-led and topic-centred seminar this may be appropriate, even if there is reason to question whether it is the best use of resources. If a learner-centred approach to the seminars is being adopted, then this needs to be made explicit by the tutor at the start of the course. If it is not made clear students may be confused and unsure of how to respond effectively in the group.

Initially, the tutor may need to suggest some guidelines as to how the group should work. This will mean encouraging students to set an agenda, for instance by listing what they hope to learn from the session. The tutor may need to help them define and focus what they really intend. It may also be important to use other group skills to ensure that everyone has an equal say in the decisions. These may include getting people to write down their personal objectives, and then sharing them. Setting an agenda, in itself, helps students at the end of a session to evaluate how successful it has been. Setting guidelines may also include ensuring that someone (other than the tutor) chairs the sessions and that someone acts as recorder. They may need to consider how time will be divided and how they may make use of any resources, including people, that are present. As students become more familiar with group-learning methods, it will be possible to increase the amount of responsibility given to students themselves to organize their own approach to meeting specified course objectives.

Problem-based learning usually imposes its own structure. Once students are used to the method (described in more detail in Chapter 14) they will quickly settle to using the trigger material to determine the areas that they should be considering in more depth, and setting their own learning objectives. The tutor, however, needs to be alert to students diverting from tasks or becoming confused, and gently lead them back to the main focus of the session. This requires interpersonal and communication skills.

Central to the development of a group must be the existence of a warm, accepting and non-threatening climate where learning is to be approached as a co-operative, rather than competitive, exercise. Group sessions and learning tasks should be enjoyable.

Whatever the format of a small group, it is essential for the tutor to have thorough understanding of and ability to apply the principles and practice of effective group learning. These include attention to various stages of the process as set out by the CVCP (Griffiths and Partington 1992):

1. *Opening*—defining the group and its purpose.
2. *Listening*—listening and encouraging students to listen to one another. What is said, when is it said, and how is it said? Was the content, the priority, and the feelings explicit? Is silence tolerated?
3. *Questioning*—an appropriate questioning style which encourages student participation. Are questions open, comprehensible, encouraging, and challenging? Is jargon and obscurity noted and understanding of participants checked?
4. *Responding*—appropriate responses to students designed to engage students and to heighten awareness of particular issues. Are interjections appropriately timed? Is silence used to encourage, build confidence, and promote thinking? Is there appropriate use of explanation, designed both to make use of the tutor's expertise, but also to identify ways of using students' experiences to provide solutions to problems.
5. *Structuring*—is there a balance between coverage of a topic and a flexible response to members needs? Are group members clear about the group direction?
6. *Closing*—is there time to round off the session and ensure that a coherent summary and plan of action has been produced?.

Tutors also require skills to handle students of different personalities and help the group to come together as a team. This includes encouragement, drawing out appropriate feelings, and even antagonism between members. Two types of student cause problems in groups: those who dominate the group, and those who have difficulty in participating. More mature groups may be able to deal with these situations themselves but sometimes tutors will have to intervene in the group process. This may be done during the group sessions themselves, or by talks with group members outside the sessions.

One way of managing these problems is for key roles within the group to be rotated. A rotating chairperson can avoid the dominant member always taking that role and can also encourage quieter members to take an active part. The position of recorder can often be used to put a person into a less dominant position during the group discussion. The group may also need to consider the strengths of individual members and this is where time spent reflecting on group process can be important. The tutor can help a group to see how the noisier members may not have brought many new ideas to the group, and that a quieter person has been effective in moving the group on either by a provocative idea, lateral thinking, or a quiet ability to summarize. Belbin (1981) described several roles that people may take in an organizational group (see Table 7.1). Many of these roles are equally applicable within an educational group. Discussion with group members can help them to see that the apparently dull and quiet member is the one who is the reliable implementer who takes the ideas of the group, turns them into action, and always has a report back available. Another group member may be an awkward communicator but, if listened to, full of creative and imaginative ideas. The best person for sorting out the goals and tasks of a group may not be the most clever or creative person.

Table 7.1   *Roles in the Group* (after Belbin 1981)

Roles	Description	Comments
Plant	Creative, imaginative, unorthodox	Weak in communicating
Resource investigator	Extrovert, enthusiastic, explores	Can lose enthusiasm
Co-Ordinator	Mature, clarifies goals, promotes decision-making	Not necessarily most clever or creative
Shaper	Challenges, pressurizes, finds way round obstacles	Prone to provocation and loss of temper
Monitor Evaluator	Sober, discerning, sees all options	Lacks drive and ability to inspire
Team-worker	Perceptive, accommodating, listens, builds, averts friction	Indecisive in crunch situations
Implementer	Disciplined, reliable, turns ideas into action	Somewhat inflexible and unresponsive to new ideas
Completer	Painstaking, anxious, searches out errors, delivers on time	Inclined to worry unduly, reluctant to delegate
Specialist	Single-minded, provides skills in rare supply	Contributes only on narrow front

THE GROUP ENVIRONMENT

A number of technical issues are likely to increase the chance of successful group work.

The right place

A comfortable room of appropriate size and without distractions should be provided. The seating should, so far as possible, be arranged to allow group members equal opportunity to contribute. This means that they need to be able to have eye contact with each other, and particularly with the chairperson. The contribution of a quiet group member may be encouraged if that person is sat opposite the chairperson, or the tutor in a tutor-led group. Conversely, an over-voluble group member can be inhibited by being sat next to the tutor. This can apply even in a learner-centred group where the closeness of the tutor has an inhibitory effect.

The right size

Groups should be of appropriate size. This is normally considered to be eight to twelve members. Smaller groups, down to three or four members may be appropriate for teaching communication skills. Groups of more than twelve are unlikely to be able to make good use of the conventional small group dynamic. If the available resources mean that such large groups are inevitable then it may be possible for them to do much of their work in two subsets. It is possible for an experienced tutor to facilitate two subsets at the same time.

The right introduction

Time should be set apart for introductions if members are not already known to each other. Introductions should involve more than exchange of names. Members should be able to share some of their background and what they hope to gain from the group. Several group-building games are available and each facilitator will probably have a favourite. The simplest involves people talking in pairs for a few minutes and then introducing their pair to the rest of the group. It is often useful to have a few basic questions to which answers are expected. These may be serious (home town, previous experience, or career hopes) or more informal (favourite music or worst moment!). Care needs to be taken to avoid the group starting in an atmosphere of mutual embarrassment.

The right rules

Groups need to be able to work to a set structure and it is important to determine the following elements:

* What are the expectations of attendance and punctuality?
* Have the length and objectives of each seminar session been established?
* Has a method of working been agreed with the group?
* Have appropriate breaks been provided?

INTERPROFESSIONAL LEARNING IN GROUPS

Medical students may be expected to gain experience of the work of other professional groups through their daily work. They may have brief one-to-one attachments but at present they rarely find themselves in a seminar room with students from other disciplines. Once qualified, doctors do not work in isolation from other disciplines. At the very least they encounter and have to communicate with other professional groups. In many branches of medicine, effective practice will depend on being able to develop effective collaboration. This is particularly true in primary care, where the operation of a primary health care team crucially depends on establishing and maintaining collaboration with a range of other workers.

The opportunity to work together with students from other health care professions in small groups is one way to promote this collaboration and to learn about communication with other disciplines and the ability to work effectively as a member of a team.

The aims of interprofessional learning should be:

- to increase knowledge and understanding of the training, roles, and skills of other professionals involved in patient care;
- to encourage interprofessional confidence and respect, and to break down stereotyped attitudes;
- to recognize common skills shared by different professions

Many of these objectives are likely to be achieved in the context of seminar teaching that involves students from more that one discipline. This may also include project work where tasks are assigned to pairs of students from different professional groups. Effective interprofessional learning is not easy to establish, not least because stereotyped attitudes are developed very early by students of most disciplines. There is also the danger that one particular profession is allowed to dominate. In many multiprofessional groups it is the doctors or medical students who tend to dominate, but it is also possible for other groups to do so. One tutor was faced with a mixed group of final-year nurses working for a Bachelor of Nursing degree, and medical students in their first clinical year. The nursing students had greater knowledge and experience of group work and this markedly inhibited the medical students who thereby failed to learn much about team-work.

However, a problem-based approach to education offers the opportunity for seminar work to be structured so that the students identify learning needs that should be addressed from the perspective of more than one discipline. One example would be the identification of roles of, for example, doctors, nurses, and physiotherapists in the management of a patient with a complex physical disability in the community. This offers the students the opportunity to mimic, in a learning situation, the co-operation which they need to develop in order to work effectively with those disciplines in the future.

A number of principles will increase the chance of developing effective interprofessional learning:

1. Learning should take place at a relatively early stage in the students' education.
2. There should be a match between the educational level of students from different professional groups.
3. Teaching sessions must be planned by staff from the relevant range of disciplines, even if a seminar is led by a tutor from one of the professions represented.
4. More than one profession should be represented among the tutors. If resources do not always allow for co-tutoring between professions, then tasks may be split. If, for example, a problem-based approach is used for the education of nurses and doctors, then either discipline could take a seminar where students identify learning needs in relation to the subject of the seminar. However, both nurses and doctors should resource the seminar where students report back on their learning experiences.

The first two principles are of the greatest importance. One of the problems of interprofessional groups in medical schools is that they are often established after that early stage, already mentioned, when students acquire stereotyped attitudes about the disciplines with whom they are then expected to work. The aim of interprofessional education is mainly to influence attitudes, and it is much more likely to be effective if it takes place at a stage before such attitudes (especially negative ones) have become ingrained.

CONCLUSION

Small groups are an effective approach to developing higher cognitive abilities such as the abilities to apply and evaluate knowledge; they are effective in developing problem-solving and communication skills and may be appropriate places to learn many practical skills. They are, above all, places where attitudes can be developed. They can promote awareness, interest and enthusiasm, and a willingness to receive and respond. They can provide the opportunity to explore values, to test out preferences and commitments, and to organize a personal value system.

Small groups are not a panacea for all educational ills. Certain questions should be answered before they are introduced to particular courses:

* Which course objectives can best be achieved within a small group setting?
* Which type of group would best achieve these objectives?
* What briefing will be required by group tutors and external resources?
* In what way should the group process be assessed and developed?

8 Lectures and laboratories

A review of educational approaches is not complete without considering more traditional formats. Community-based tutors are less likely to be involved in giving lectures or providing demonstrations and supervision in laboratories. However, there will be occasions when a lecture may be used to introduce a concept. The development of what are termed 'skills laboratories' may also provide opportunities for tutors from the community to participate in teaching basic clinical and communication skills in a new way.

THE USE OF LECTURES

The lecture format has been most frequently used in medical schools as a method of conveying factual knowledge, however, it is not necessarily effective at this. Although the best lectures can provide an inspired introduction to large numbers of students, the worst can have a negative effect on students' interest in and appreciation of a subject. With the availability of technology to lecture to larger and larger groups, including students in different parts of the country by videolink, it is important that lectures should be delivered by lecturers with the greatest skill and understanding of how the lecture format can be used as a basis for active learning.

Changes in medical education, and particularly education in the community, have placed greater emphasis on the development of skills and attitudes rather than knowledge. In general, the lecture format is less suitable for achieving these aims, although a lecture can motivate rethinking about values and attitudes or the need to develop a skill.

Despite these disadvantages, there are some situations where the lecture will be the method of choice. These include:

- providing an introduction to or overview of a subject to a large group of students;
- providing up-to-date information about the advancing edge of a topic, including the latest research;
- initiating discussion about a controversial topic including an ethical issue;
- inspiring interest and motivation through hearing key workers in a field.

A wide range of community related topics are amenable to introduction in lecture format, from the roles and functions of members of the primary care team to the importance of communication skills and discussion of patients' rights. The lecture may initiate some surface learning that can then be augmented by deeper integrative learning through the wide range of teaching methods described earlier.

THE TECHNIQUE OF LECTURING

The traditional lecture consists of a lecture reading a structured talk for 40 minutes to 1 hour from a podium, possibly with some use of visual aids such as an overhead projector or slides. This may not be suited to students who are used to a more visual and quick-moving presentation of information, as is found on television, nor to those who have been trained to be more active in their learning. The subject matter alone is not enough to win an audience. Some basic technical points need attention for any successful lecture. Care needs to be given to the following.

Preparation and delivery

The material to be presented must be carefully prepared. Very few lecturers, even the most experienced, can deliver an effective lecture which has not been very carefully planned. If a script is being used then it also requires practise so that it does not appear as if it is being read AND fits comfortably within the time slot available.

The delivery must be clear so that people can hear what is said without straining. Consideration must be given to the volume and the articulation. If a microphone is available, it should be used unless the speaker is absolutely sure that the voice carries to the back of the hall when it is full. If the microphone is fixed, then it is important to find the right, comfortable position from which to speak and note any movement that affects the sound. Attention must be paid to the speed of speaking and avoiding a voice that drops at the end of a sentence: both of these are common faults, often ascribed to nervousness.

Visual aids

Effective visual aids need not be very sophisticated. The art is in producing material which is visually attractive and makes the point as concisely as possible. This may vary from videoclips, through slides to overhead transparencies or even the use of a whiteboard (in a smaller room). The essential feature is that visual aids must be visible! They must be able to be seen from all parts of the room, and they must be readable (if there is text) and audible (if a videoclip is being shown).

Videoclips may be a particularly effective way of enhancing an introductory lecture on a subject such as communication skills. They can also be used to introduce a patient's view into a lecture on ethics. Suitable clips may be found in television documentaries, or even in medical soap operas. Copyright must be considered but universities will often have permission and facilities for 'off-air' recording for educational purposes. The lecturer needs to be absolutely certain that the equipment will perform to the standard needed. Many an introduction has been spoilt by a high-pitched feedback hum.

Highly sophisticated equipment is now available for the projection of computer-generated images: however, five lines on a simple overhead transparency is infinitely better than an illegible multimedia presentation or one which does not work at all. Overhead transparencies have several advantages over slides or projected images. The room does not need to be darkened and it is easier for the lecturer to maintain an interaction with the audience. It is possible to build up a presentation by using overlays. This is preferable to slowly uncovering parts of an transparency, as the covers invariably become untidy or fall off at the wrong moment and the students are always more interested in what is hidden than what is shown. It is possible to draw or add words during the presentation as long as one is able to do this neatly and legibly.

However, if using transparencies, certain rules need to be considered. Only certain colours are easily visible. Blue is best, followed by black and green. Red is very difficult and yellow usually impossible. Transparencies should also contain restricted amounts of information. In preparing either overheads or slides, it is worth following the 'rule of eights' (Box 1)

Effective time use

It is important to limit the length of a lecture. Concentration starts to fall after 20 minutes, and falls sharply after 40 minutes. Lectures should be structured to take account of the attention span. This includes having a number of points to introduce at intervals. It also means using intermediate summaries and appropriate visual aids. It is often helpful to have a slide of the aims of the lecture and to use it to remind the audience what point has been reached. Some of the techniques described below can be used to break up a long lecture in order to keep the concentration of the audience.

If the lecturer wants to make further key points at the end of an hour's lecture then specific attention must be paid to how to recapture the attention of the flagging audience. Variation in pace and style of delivery can also help. If the microphones and acoustics of the room allow, this can include change of position. Humour, whether verbal or visual (e.g. cartoons), is commonly used. This can be an effective way of producing breaks in delivery style, although the lecturer needs to be careful to avoid humour which might offend and even alienate sections of the audience. There is no place for humour that might be considered sexist, racist, or obscene. Care must also be taken about anecdotes or cartoons that belittle other disciplines or health professions.

Box 1   The rule of eights

For slides and overhead transparencies:
• EIGHT words a line
• EIGHT lines on a slide
• Visible at a distance of EIGHT screen diagonals

Handout

Handouts have various purposes. They can be used to provide an overview of the lecture on which students can take more detailed notes. They can be used to provide a summary of the lecture with ideas for further reading or work to be done.

Handouts to be used as prior overviews can be circulated at the start of a lecture, but are better presented in advance with the students' course material. Such handouts risk reducing the spontaneity of the lecture. There is also a danger that students will read the handout rather than listen to the lecture. They should therefore not attempt to provide a complete summary of a lecture: they should rather be used as a guide to the student. With some of the more modern computer programs for making overhead transparencies or slides it is possible to provide reductions of the slides with space for the student to make additional notes.

Handouts are not a quick way to guarantee information transfer: indeed they can fall foul of the adage that information passes 'from the notes of the lecturer to the notes of the student without passing through the mind of either'. However, used in the right way, they can be an effective adjunct to orient the student to the lecture material and to provide a summary of the content.

Handouts provided at the end of the lecture should also not be a mere summary of the information provided. This risks students coming at the end to collect the handout, rather than at the beginning to hear the lecturer. They can provide a summary of a framework which the lecturer has built up and they can provide ideas for further discussion or exploration and suggestions how the lecture information might be used. In a series of lectures they can also be used to suggest tasks and activities to be undertaken before the next of the series.

ACTIVE LEARNING IN THE LECTURE THEATRE

At first sight, lecture theatres are the epitome of passive learning. However, it is possible for a lecturer faced with 150 students in a lecture theatre to apply the principles of active learning and thereby maximize the impact of the lecture. The principles are the same as those which underlay active learning in other situations: students need the opportunity to think reflect and discuss. Several active learning techniques can be applied specifically to lectures.

Questions

The lecturer can ask questions of the students. The questions should be real ones (i.e. not just questions with predetermined answers designed to shift the focus away from the lecturer for a brief time). Closed questions are unlikely to stimulate thought. However, open questions risk not getting a response at all in a large lecture theatre. It is helpful if the question is presented on an overhead slide, though the lecturer must retain flexibility in the use of questions during his or her lecture. The lecturer may ask if clarification is needed after the students have had a short time to think. In order to ensure responses, students can be asked to write down their answer, or to discuss it with a neighbour. The lecturer should avoid humiliating students by directing difficult questions at one person in a large group.

The lecturer can encourage questions from the students. It needs to be made clear at the start of a lecture if students are being encouraged to interrupt. If the lecturer wishes to use this format, it is helpful to provide brief pauses from time to time during which the lecturer may remind students that they can ask questions.

Brainstorming

Brainstorming can be used as a way of including the views of a wide range of students. As students call out ideas, the lecturer writes these on an overhead transparency or a board. As with questions from the lecturer, students may need to be given a time to think and write suggestions down in order to ensure a response from the audience.

'Buzz groups'

These groups can be used to enable students to take an active part in discussing material which has been presented by the lecturer. The students arrange themselves in groups of two or three for this activity, which is quite feasible even in a banked lecture theatre.

Two or three buzz groups can be asked to summarize their conclusions, gradually increasing the combined size of the group until it is possible for a small number of groups to feed back to the whole lecture theatre. This technique, the *progressive group*, is particularly effective for handling controversial subjects.

Lecturers can be afraid that the situation will run riot once students are allowed out of their strait-jacket of polite silence but it is possible to keep control, even in a large theatre, without raising voices. The dimmer switch can be a very effective method of bringing attention back to the lecturer.

THE 'SKILLS LABORATORY'

A recent development in medical schools has been the development of skills laboratories. This has provided the possibility for resources relating to a learning a range of skills to be centralized. These resources include:

- Manikins on which basic examination and practical skills can be practised. Fundoscopy, auscultation, rectal and vaginal examination, venepuncture, and suturing can all be practised using equipment of this nature, much of which is now highly sophisticated and realistic.
- Audiovisual facilities for communication-skills teaching. This will include rooms, cameras and recording equipment, and also simulated patients.

The impetus for development of skills laboratories related partly to the increasing difficulty in using in-patients for teaching, partly to the recognition that it is ethically unacceptable for groups of students to carry out painful or embarrassing procedures on patients, and partly to the development of materials which may substitute for real patients in some situations. They provide an opportunity to structure teaching so that it is available when required by students, they also offer opportunities for the assessment of students under set conditions. For instance, standardized simulated patients may be used in order to provide a standardized method of assessing students' communication skills.

The development of interactive computer-based learning and virtual reality technology are likely to increase substantially the opportunities for new technologies to contribute to medical student education in the future.

Community-based tutors will be able to interact with these new learning facilities in many ways. They may be asked to run sessions on specific skills for a group of students. Although skills laboratories provide an extra resource for active learning, they do not do away with the need for a live tutor on many occasions. This is particularly true in learning communication and examination skills. General practitioners, with their long experience in communication training, will have a particular expertise to offer here. Community-based tutors also need to be aware of these facilities as they develop and be prepared to direct students to them. A student who is inept at using an otoscope or carrying out a venepuncture could be advised to sign up for further remedial sessions in a skills laboratory.

Many medical schools may not opt for a purpose-built skills laboratory such as that at Maastricht. On the other hand they may arrange for the materials to be available at several bases (which could include larger community teaching centres as well as hospitals).

CONCLUSION

Traditional approaches, such as lectures, will continue to have a valuable role in medical education. Tutors asked to participate need to ensure that their input is relevant to an audience that is likely to be used to a more active approach to learning. Community tutors also need to be aware of newer approaches to education. Clinical learning is no longer divided solely between the hospital and the community, the advent of skills laboratories provides a new structured approach to acquiring many skills.

9 Choosing an approach

A wide range of educational approaches has now been explored. The next stage is to consider how to use them effectively to meet the educational objectives of students and tutors. The approach should be tailored to promote the most effective use of the time and resources available and to cope with the varied needs of the students. The following chapters review a number of different areas identified in Chapter 4 where learning objectives in the community were discussed. For each area, different educational approaches are considered to demonstrate how the objectives might be achieved. Clearly, some objectives (such as learning about the individual, the family, and assessment of patients) can and should be achieved concurrently. To avoid undue repetition the areas chosen bring together a number of objectives and methods. Even so, the limited number of broad approaches means some repetition is inevitable, but the examples given show how methods can be adapted to meet different needs. This will provide a compendium of ideas, not for imitation but to stimulate educational problem-solving when faced with questions of how to facilitate an area of learning.

A number of factors should influence a decision to use a particular method. These include:

Course factors:
- Time available.
- Position within curriculum.
- Integration with other aspects of the course.
- Size of learning groups.
- The designated assessment methods.
- The timing of assessments.

Student factors:
- Age.
- Previous educational experience.
- Personal aims and ambitions.
- Existence of known remedial needs.
- Attitudes and motivation.

Resource factors:
- Training and experience of tutors.

- Commitment of tutors from other disciplines and professions.
- The cost of resource people.
- Availability of facilities such as interview or seminar rooms.
- Availability of equipment such as recording systems.
- Availability of information resources such as libraries.

Some examples will show how important these factors may be in tailoring an educational approach.

Integration of course

One tutor is seldom entirely responsible for planning the learning of a student. In vocational training a general practitioner trainer may be responsible for setting a learning plan for a full year, but even here the task is shared with the course organizer and is related to the learning that takes place in other posts during the training period. In undergraduate training a single tutor is likely to be concerned with only a small part of the course. That period of learning has to be integrated with the rest of the course. If it is not it may appear irrelevant and is likely to be less effectively learnt. A totally strange approach to learning may disorientate students and make it less likely that they feel fully involved. On the other hand, a new approach properly explained and negotiated can enthuse students and thereby promote their learning.

Training factors

Other people working with a tutor as co-tutors or resources must understand the objectives and the educational methods being used so that they work in the same way. There is a frequent problem when students are encouraged to develop self-learning and questioning methods. A session with a resource practitioner is arranged and the students prepare a series of questions in advance. At the session the first question is met with a prepared speech complete with illustrative slides, handouts, and leaflets that cover the visitor's objectives, but not necessarily those of the students who feel that preparation time has been wasted.

Many people who are willing to act as resources will not have been trained in educational method. They anticipate they are expected to have materials prepared and go to considerable trouble to do this. They arrive anxious to put over their message. This previously prepared material gives them confidence that they will not omit salient points. It is impolite and unkind not to allow them to use this. Time must be devoted to prior briefing and methods must be chosen that make the best use of their skills and expertise, and often limited time.

Assessment factors

It is natural for student minds to be focused on assessment. They have lived with the concept of regular hurdles for many years and perceive courses as steeple-chases rather than flat racing. They will choose learning objectives that relate to the assessments.

This point is developed in Part V. Well-planned assessments will take account of this and make sure key objectives are not forgotten. A good example of this was the change in assessment methods at Southampton (Coles 1990) where, in a traditional two-part curriculum, preclinical assessment was delayed until students had done a year of the clinical course. This encouraged students to integrate their knowledge of basic sciences with clinical knowledge. Those who used revision approaches that did this fared better.

However, there will be times in all courses when students will be concerned about forthcoming assessments that may seem irrelevant to the objectives of the current session or block. In these circumstances it may be possible to choose a learning approach that has a dual purpose: it prepares the students for their assessment while fulfilling other objectives at the same time. One tutor was asked to provide a morning session on the subject of 'ethics and clinical problem-solving' immediately prior to the written part of Finals. Other topics in the lecture course ranged from the acute abdomen to obstetric complications. Although the Finals examination included patient-management problems, the ethical aspects were not included in the marking schedule. The solution was to run a symposium that presented a series of patient-management problems in the fields of obstetrics, geriatrics, surgery, and oncology, and to help the students to consider questions such as 'To examine or not to examine (vaginally)', 'To investigate or not to investigate (in an elderly patient)' 'To tell or not to tell (before surgery)', and 'To treat or not to treat (an inoperable cancer)'. In this way, students were encouraged to think wider than the clinical management, but were not totally diverted from their main concerns at the time.

Resources

Facilities and equipment influence the choice of approach. The use of videorecording requires good equipment which is easily set up and which has simple controls. Again, choices need to be made between the use of real patients or other resources, such as standardized patients or student role-play, when working in a field such as communication. A properly trained 'patient—tutor' can be expensive. To use such a skilled resource for simple history-taking experience would be inappropriate.

CONCLUSION

The choice of a suitable approach can be a difficult task. The approaches suggested in the following chapters are by no means comprehensive. They are intended to show how skills and resources can be adapted to the purpose in hand. They will show how different teaching methods can address the same objectives in an attempt to deal with the wide needs of students working in the community setting. It is quite wrong to believe that the close one-to-one tutorial, as effective as it is, can address effectively all these needs. There are no doubt many other examples that could be given. Some are provided in Part IV. However, with any approach the following questions should be asked:

- Are the student's learning needs known?
- Are objectives for a particular session or period clear?
- Is the chosen method appropriate to those objectives?
- How will the success of the approach be evaluated?

10 Learning how to assess the needs of a population

Important public health areas of population medicine can be taught in a community setting and even within individual general practices. This is especially true in the United Kingdom where practices are responsible for a defined population. The development of computerized records now means that practices have access to more data about their populations. This is being increasingly used to plan services. It is also available for students to learn simple epidemiological skills. Planning of services also requires knowledge of whether a problem is prevalent and whether a proposed solution is effective. Skills in the critical assessment of evidence about the value of investigations and managements is therefore required. This leads students into the whole field of clinical epidemiology. This chapter will consider the use of lectures, projects, and multiprofessional learning in gaining these skills.

LECTURES

Assessment of needs requires understanding of the basic principles of epidemiology and of population surveys. It also requires some ability to work with statistics. Some of these skills can be learnt from resources, such as books, but a lecture course may provide a useful framework as well as direct students to available resources. This field has traditionally been the preserve of public health departments, but other community staff will increasingly contribute to the field, especially as clinical epidemiological skills are needed.

Suitable objectives.

In a lecture students can learn:

- to understand the nature of populations;
- to understand the basic principles of epidemiology;
- basic statistical methods for population research.

Students will gain more from a lecture by being given some preparation work. They can be asked to describe the population in a practice to which they are attached. They may be able to obtain an age—sex histogram from the computer. They may look for local census information that will show them the ethnic or occupational mix of the area. They should compare their population to the national average. This exercise should help them to consider how a population that is younger, older, poorer, or more ethnically variable will have different health needs. It will also give them an insight into the paucity of information on which many a practice profile is based. Most practices can produce little more than an age—sex register.

The lecture itself can build on the preparation. In the example above it might consider widely different populations and explore how these differences might affect the services that were needed. The lecturer can then explore some of the difficulties in assessing the population needs. Interactive methods, such as 'buzz groups', can be used when there has been preparatory work. The lecturer can encourage students to continue reflecting on the issues by ending with some tasks to carry out in their own practice. One instance would be to do a sample of attenders and to discern how representative this was of the practice area. There are other possibilities which may well lead into a project (see below).

MULTIPROFESSIONAL AND MULTIDISCIPLINARY LEARNING

Many people are involved in assessing needs. A nurse will have a different concept of the needs of the population to that of a doctor. Similarly, a public health doctor looking at the wide population of a district will have a different approach to a general practitioner with a registered list of patients. It is in this area that multidisciplinary and multiprofessional learning can help students understand that different approaches are complementary and not antagonistic.

Suitable objectives

With multidisciplinary input students can learn:

- to understand the range of assessments that can be made;
- skills in the resolution of conflicts about needs;
- to respect the inputs of different professionals.

In the previous chapters, learning with other disciplines was considered in terms of shared learning between different professions (see p.77). Here a different range of resources may be of help to the student. Different medical disciplines may discuss how they assess needs. As the students explore the approaches of these disciplines they will discover some conflicts. They should explore the value systems on which these are based and how these can positively enhance a proper debate about needs.

A seminar might be resourced by representatives from public health, general practice, and other disciplines such as community paediatrics, geriatrics, or occupational medicine. The needs of the elderly within the practice might be a suitable subject. Preparatory work by the students would help them consider the needs of elderly patients in a broad way (from rehabilitation and social support to medical care) and what resources are provided. They might collect information on particular resources such as waiting lists for hip operations and cataracts. In the seminar discussion, public health physicians can show how they allocate resources for services, such as a cataract extraction service, and clinicians can show how they assess the needs of individual patients, and seek to achieve the best service for them. The students should be allowed to reflect on the different approaches and have time to discuss the reasons and effects of these.

PROJECT

One of the most effective ways of helping students to learn about population needs in the mini-population of a practice is to give them the opportunity to do a small data-collecting project as the first stage of an audit cycle. The increased availability of computer information enables much of this to be done fairly simply and students are usually familiar with necessary information technology skills such as use of spreadsheets. Students may wish to add a record review or a series of interviews with a selected group of patients.

Suitable objectives

Through a project students can learn:

- skills of data collection and interpretation;
- sampling methods;
- questionnaire design and administration;
- evaluation and application of population data.

In approaching a project, students should choose a subject where there is a reasonable sample of patients. All patients of a particular age may be chosen and an analysis done of their morbidity. Patients with a particular condition may be chosen and a survey done of the services and treatment they are receiving. For less common conditions all the patients in the practice might be sampled and interviewed.

EXAMPLE 1

One student decided to sample 20% of the practice patients with asthma and to follow-up a record review with a questionnaire to determine their current state of health. It was possible from the records to discover what proportion had peak flow rates recorded. It was also possible to use the peak flow rates as a marker of success of treatment. The questionnaire provided a picture of the patients' self-perception of their health status. This could be compared with the peak flow rates and an evaluation made of any need for a change in services.

EXAMPLE 2

Another student looked at knowledge and use of the drug 'Ecstasy' among a population identified by contact in a contact-tracing approach. People who had been occasional or regular users were then asked about their use of primary health care services, and their perceptions of general practitioners. The study threw light on why patients needs may not be recognized.

EXAMPLE 3

A third student studied how many patients failed to have their prescriptions dispensed. By following up a record review of these patients the study threw light on the likelihood that doctors sometimes perceive a need (for a prescription) that is not perceived by the patient.

Further examples of projects are given by Blackie and Campion in Chapter 25.

11 Learning about the family

In Chapter 4 the concept of the family was considered in social, psychological, and genetic terms and the influence of the family on health discussed. The community is the main setting in which this influence and its significance can be discovered.

There are difficulties in achieving educational objectives related to the family partly because students arrive with their own preconceptions. Everyone knows what a family is until that understanding is shaken by an encounter with a totally different, but equally valid alternative. Exposure to a range of cultures and societies shows that there is a wide variation of family structure. Only a minority of patients experience a traditional nuclear family. Students should be encouraged to discover the scope of households and family structures and to consider the implications. They will need to include different constructs of the family that include:

- lone parent families, nuclear families, and extended families;
- various types of partnership including reconstituted partnership and same-sex partnership;
- households of one, two, or three generations;
- sharing families and separated families (i.e. those families that share the same house, the same few streets, or the same culture, and those families separated by hundreds of miles physically or emotionally).

All these aspects can affect health and health care. The doctor has to learn to move beyond the genogram and to work with a wide team in responding to all these influences, especially when dealing with the new generations arriving and the previous generations departing.

There are many opportunities in the community setting for students to experience and reflect on the influence of the family.

PRIMARY HEALTH CARE TEAM ATTACHMENTS

The involvement of different professionals means that students can learn through attachments to others in the primary care team.

Suitable objectives

When attached to primary health care team members students can learn to:

- understand the range of family structures in society;
- understand how a team approach can promote the health of a family;
- accept a wide range of social backgrounds and cultures.

The most important attachment for these objectives will be with a health visitor, although within the primary care team, students may also spend time with nurses and midwives. Opportunities can also be taken for placements with other workers in the community such as social workers or link workers. An attachment to a link worker, involved with patients from ethnic minorities, can be very important in helping students gain insights into the family structures and needs of patients from other cultures.

Occasionally there will be the opportunity for attachment to someone who is specified as a 'family worker', or alternatively to workers with particular age groups, such as youth workers or a visitor to the elderly, who may have considerable insights into the way families affect health needs. The planning of an attachment with a health visitor is provided as an example of how these learning opportunities should be managed.

The health visitor attachment

The health visitor's role theoretically covers all age groups, although in many areas this role has become limited to families with young children. In some areas, there may be the opportunity to meet health visitors with other defined responsibilities (e.g. to the elderly, to children with disabilities, or to homeless families).

The health visitor's role includes:

- assessment of community, family, and individual needs;
- co-ordination and delivery of preventive services (e.g. immunization);
- co-ordination and delivery of screening and surveillance services (e.g. child health surveillance);
- providing health promotion and advice, especially to families with infants.

Some of these roles will be further discussed in the chapter on health promotion.

Planning experience with health visitors needs to be carefully managed. It should include clinical contacts with families and avoid the detailed administrative work. Clinical contact can be arranged in a child health clinic, or during the domiciliary work carried out by health visitors. Time for discussion and reflection should be arranged, even if it is limited to time spent together in a car.

Students may not realize the importance of the time spent with a health visitor. The experience may be dominated by advice on baby-management and social security benefits. The health visitor's role in the identification and alleviation of family stress can be overlooked. Health visitors are usually very willing to take medical students with them for a session and to talk about their training and roles, but much of this can be lost unless the students are prepared in advance to make the best use of the time. What the health visitor has to impart must be linked to what the students need to learn. In group work or tutorials with their tutor students should have worked out their learning objectives, and prepared appropriate questions. Health visitors should be briefed to explore these with the students. A consultation with a mother where there was a language barrier, or a refusal to receive an immunization, can trigger appropriate questions on family structure and influence that can be discussed with health visitors.

Students also need to consider how to make use of time spent with the health visitor on home visits. Often during the visit there may only be one parent and one or two children at home. The influence of the other parent, of children at school and of the extended family may be important. Students should reflect on their expectations prior to the visit, making use of any prior knowledge they have through previous contact or records. They can then discuss differences between expectations and actuality with the health visitor.

INDEPENDENT VISITS

Several medical schools have conducted family attachment schemes for students for many years (see the description by McGlade in Chapter 16). These attachments may start in the first year of the medical course. Students then have the opportunity to visit a family on a number of occasions over months or years to see how that family copes with a life event or health problem. A family can be identified when a birth is expected within six to eight weeks. The students can then visit that family before the birth and at a number of times after the birth and look at the process of a adjustment, the health beliefs, the needs, and the health care input. Such early patient contact can be very influential for students but the learning objectives should be clear.

Suitable objectives.

On independent visits and attachments students can learn:

* the structure and relationships within a family;
* the ideas, concerns, and expectations of a family;
* the coping strategies of a family;
* the perceptions of the health services of different family members.
* skills in building relationships with different family members.

A successful independent attachment requires depth of involvement and length of contact. The student should not restrict their involvement to one easily accessible person (e.g. the expectant mother). To meet the mother of a new baby has value in learning aspects of adjusting to a new child but only gives a monocular view of the family. To understand the structure and relationships and to discover also how ideas concerns and expectations evolve, students should meet as many family members as possible. Any resident partner should be included and, if possible, close relatives who visit regularly such as grandparents and siblings.

Attitudes and concerns change over time: a great advantage of a family attachment is to watch the process by which different members adapt to the life event or illness. Students should note down concerns or uncertainties that family members have during a particular visit. On a later visit they should review whether these concerns remain and, if not, how they have been resolved.

Shorter family visits can be important. In the community follow-up of patients discharged from hospital one objective should always to be to talk to the carers of the patient as the following example shows:

EXAMPLE 1

A student had seen a patient with a myocardial infarct discharged from hospital. She had heard the advice given to the patient on rehabilitation. She had seen how that had been confirmed in leaflets. Later a visit was made to the patient at home. His mobility had decreased since he had left hospital. His wife had not been given any advice and her concern for her partner had meant that she had waited on him hand and foot and not allowed him to do anything, even walk into the garden or make himself a cup of tea.

Precautions need to be taken about family visits and attachments. Especially on longer attachments, students can be drawn in to the family circle. They can then be asked for advice or help which they do not yet have the knowledge or experience to give. Students need to be aware of this and helped to learn strategies to divert the request. They may act as advocates (reporting the concern to a health care professional), but need to beware of advising beyond their competence. A further danger is that they may become involved in family disagreements, and feel that they are being asked to take sides. This can be distressing. A tutor should be available to debrief students after visits to their family.

PROJECTS

A family attachment gives a view of a single family. However, if several students carry out family attachments at the same time, this experience can be extended. This can be done formally with structured questionnaires and collation of the results and then form the basis of a group project as in the 'Family Study' developed at Newcastle upon Tyne (see the contribution by Drinkwater in McCrorie *et al.* 1993).

Suitable objectives

Through a project, students can learn:

- an understanding of survey methods available in behavioural sciences;
- skill in formal and informal questioning and the differences between them;
- the range of structures of families and attitudes displayed by families;
- how to evaluate material provided in social science surveys and to apply the research when dealing with individuals;

Group projects, like the 'Family Study' require a reasonably sized group of students. Students will need to consider what response rates they are expecting and how many families they can contact. A small group of students will be able to design their own questionnaire, but will have to accept that in the time available to them they will not be able to interview enough families to do more than a pilot survey. Alternatively, a larger group (a year group) can agree to use a standardized questionnaire produced either by tutors or by some of their peers. This questionnaire can be used to collect data on a much larger sample of families, and all students can have access to the material from this data. One compromise is to use a standard questionnaire to which each group (or even student) adds a few extra questions to illuminate an area of particular interest.

A project of this nature gives students first-hand experience of social science research and ethics, although this objective about families is one of many under which social survey methodology can be learnt. Students learn the difficulties of structured, or semi-structured interviews. They learn the importance of completing a structured questionnaire in a structured way, and not on the basis of the remembered parts of an informal interview. They also need to consider issues of confidentiality as applied to interviews and to the results of the questionnaire.

However, the purpose of the project is to achieve certain objectives such as learning about the family. Students need to reflect individually on the findings and their implications for individual families. This evaluation should be included in the discussion section of the report and should be the basis for a considerable portion of the feedback. Restriction of feedback to the scientific methodology may inhibit the learning of the students.

12 Learning about health promotion and prevention

Health care has always been concerned with the maintenance of health as much as the treatment of illness. Many of the great anecdotes of 19th-century medicine, such as the story of John Snow and the Broad Street pump, relate to the maintenance of people's health. In the outbreak of cholera that swept through London in 1854, Snow plotted the geographical location of each case and implicated the water supply from a particular pump in Broad Street. By having the handle of the pump removed the (already declining) epidemic was brought to an end. However, for many years Aesculapius has overshadowed Hygeia: in other words, the focus on diagnosis and treatment has overshadowed preventive health care and health promotion.

Now the wheel is turning. Medical care has become ever more expensive. Although there have been phenomenal achievements in overcoming many infectious illness, new scourges have appeared. The devastation of degenerative illness has come to the fore. The need for health promotion has again become evident. As was seen in Chapter 1, this has become a major theme in the changes in health care and in medical education. An unresolved question is the extent of knowledge and skills that a doctor needs in this field. Many other workers are involved in health promotion. Many aspects of public health and health education may require comparatively little medical input as compared with input from environmental health officers and health promotion workers.

The community, however, remains the place to learn about concepts of health and how it is measured and maintained. Medical students need to be aware of the risk-taking behaviour of patients and of the need for prevention of disease and disability at different levels. They need to consider different attitudes of both patients and professionals to health promotion. They need to learn about the different professionals involved in health promotion, together with their respective skills. Finally, they need to evaluate the role of doctors in the promotion of health.

PRIMARY HEALTH CARE TEAM ATTACHMENTS

Other members of the primary health care team, such as health visitors, have always had health promotion high on their agenda. More recently, especially since the 1990 contract changed the terms of service to include health promotion and disease prevention within the definition of General Medical Services, general practice has been encouraged to take a greater role in relation to health promotion. One aspect of this has been the development of the role of the practice nurse. Practice nurses have developed high levels of skill in this area and many activities are now devolved to them.

Suitable objectives

Attachments to members of the primary health care team can enable students to learn:

- the basic approaches to the promotion of the health of individuals including education, immunization, and screening;
- the skills which can motivate people to a healthy lifestyle;
- the range of attitudes to health promotion.

The students need to spend time with the two team members mentioned: health visitors and practice nurses.

Health visitor attachment

The value of an attachment to the health visitor in learning about families has already been discussed in Chapter 11. Here, the use of the same attachment to achieve a different objective is considered. The planned, preventive care provided by a health visitor, is scarcely seen in hospital settings and so it is important for students to learn about the valuable role of health visitors in preventive child health services and in health education of families with small children.

For almost 150 years, health visitors have been involved in visiting people to help them consider aspects of their lifestyles that would promote their health. The student who does a series of visits with a health visitor will see how that worker builds up a relationship, discusses the patient's perceptions and needs, and relates their advice and information to those perceptions. Even though health visitors concentrate on the care of mothers with children under the age of 5 there are many different aspects that will be discussed: the effects of diet (of mother and child), the effects of smoking, the need for immunization, and the question of contraception, are all areas that will be brought up on a single visiting round. Prior preparation includes asking the student to consider the health needs of a young mother. This should make the student reflect on the essential nature of health. As with other attachments these preparatory considerations should be followed by observation and a chance to debrief effectively.

Practice nurse attachment

Practices will organize health promotion in different ways. The particular value of general practice is the responsibility for a population of patients (the practice list) and the one-to-one contacts. The organization of population initiatives, such as screening recall programmes, should be considered. Students should also be able to consider the effectiveness of personal knowledge and contact in facilitating changes in lifestyle and the need to promote health in an individual and social context. Practice nurses are commonly involved in a number of aspects: the registration health checks, annual visits to the elderly, diabetes and asthma clinics, and areas such as stress management or stopping smoking clinics. In these, a wide range of skills is displayed in promoting the health of individuals.

Students should consider what role a practice nurse might have, follow this up by observation and then evaluate this. Students should have the opportunity to reflect on the way that the nurses work is organized and how that might reflect the importance of the health-promotion agenda. Students also need to evaluate what is done. They may too easily accept that procedures are proven and acceptable. Attachments with practice nurses should be used to encourage them to take a more critical approach. They need to assess the evidence for regular cervical cytology or routine cholesterol checks.

SMALL-GROUP LEARNING

The assessment of the evidence may require the more critical atmosphere of small-group work. Small groups can also help students to take a more broad-based approach to health promotion, so that they do not focus down to, for example, the one track of 'STOP SMOKING'.

Suitable objectives:

In small-group sessions the students can learn:

- a broad range of health promotion activities in the community;
- to assess and evaluate the health promotion activities of a practice;
- motivational skills for health promotion;
- to explore their own attitudes to health promotion within medical practice.

A small-group session on health promotion might be triggered by a description of a patient seen in the community setting. This might be a patient attending for a health check. Students should be encouraged to take a broad view of how people's health can be promoted. Initial comments will often be limited to direct lifestyle changes such as smoking and alcohol consumption. Students need to be prompted to consider the barriers to success in this field. Next, students will tend to think of clinical procedures such as screening and immunization. They need to consider the evidence for screening procedures, and to learn the criteria that should be considered before introducing a screening test. The following should now be considered (Donaldson and Donaldson 1993):

1. Is the disease an important health problem?
2. Is there a recognizable latent or early symptomatic stage?
3. Are facilities for diagnosis and treatment available?
4. Has the cost of the programme been considered in the context of other demands?
5. Is there an agreed policy on whom to treat as patients?
6. Does treatment confer benefit?

These considerations will enable them to comment rationally on proposed procedures. They may need prompting to consider wider aspects such as finance and housing, exercise and nutrition, coping with stress, or sexual health.

Having considered the possible approaches, the next stage is to compare and evaluate. Examples of questions that might be asked include what approaches would be most effective in reduction of HIV infection or whether taxation or health education is the best way to reduce tobacco consumption. In these discussions, a health promotion worker or public health doctor may be a useful resource.

Small groups also provide the opportunity to evaluate the health promotion activities of a practice against a wider canvas. Members might explore the range of attitudes that abound in practices (from enthusiast to cynic) and at the same time explore and re-evaluate their own attitudes.

Finally, discussions may encourage members to acquire more effective skills for motivating people to change their lifestyle or promote their own health. This might be done by the use of role-play within a group session.

ONE-TO-ONE TEACHING

Students may see health promotion as something that other people do, whether health promotion officers or practice nurses. They need to explore and evaluate the role of a doctor in this field and how health promotion can be included within the context of every day work. This can be done within the one-to-one attachments to a GP tutor.

Suitable objectives

In the one-to-one tutorial relationship the student can learn:

- to understand the role of the individual practitioner in health promotion;
- to understand the opportunities that exist for individual health promotion;
- to assess a patient's motivation to consider health promotion;
- positive attitudes to health promotion.

During an individual surgery session the student can log the different opportunities for health promotion that were seen and whether these opportunities were taken. One surgery might have the following opportunities:

- the smoker with a cough,
- the overweight patient with pains in the knees,
- the young girl requesting contraceptive advice
- the drug addict who might benefit from hepatitis B vaccination.

If the student is logging these opportunities it will be possible to discuss reasons why they were not grasped. In the logging process, students should also consider whether the patient seemed to respond to any approach that was made. This should lead to a discussion of the health beliefs and the locus of control of patients. Finally, the student should be encouraged to take a critical look at the attitudes amongst doctors. Having reflected on these aspects students will be able to explore their own feelings about health-promotion activity within the context of medical practice, as against the broader context of health care in a population.

13 Learning about disease, illness, and treatment

This might be considered the central theme of medical education. When objectives in these fields were considered, it became clear that a community setting could greatly assist people to take a broader approach. This applied to the range of problems, the range of solutions, and the range of therapists. Students need to consider problems in clinical, individual, and contextual terms. They need to learn how to develop management plans in the same three areas and to reflect on the team-work that would facilitate this. These are the particular territory of general practice. In this chapter, methods of achieving this broader outlook will be considered through two particular areas: disability and dying. This will be followed by a consideration of a key element in extending the care of sick people: the primary health care team.

LEARNING ABOUT DISABILITY AND HANDICAP

Disability, as the word itself implies, relates to what people are able to do. Within the protected environment of an institution it is not always clear that people are unable to carry out a particular function. It is the responsibility of care providers to check such disabilities before patients are discharged.

Handicap relates to people's function within their social milieu. It is therefore especially concerned with the contextual aspects of diagnosis and management. The extent of handicap cannot be easily discovered away from that normal milieu. Learning the extent to which disabilities handicap people necessitates experience within communities. Within communities they can learn various aspects:

(1) how handicap can be overcome, either by helping the person or changing the environment;
(2) the feasibility of changes;
(3) the wide team of workers that is required;
(4) above all, that reduction of handicap requires divergent thinking and the ability to stand away from narrow medical models.

One-to-one teaching in practices provides insight into the effects of disability and multiprofessional seminars provide opportunities to explore available options. However, this section looks at three key ways of helping students learn about handicap.

INDEPENDENT VISITS

The best way for students to discover about individual and contextual aspects of assessing problems and to learn what effect a disabling illness has on the life of a patient and a household, is for them to spend time in that household. This is particularly true when people have chronic disabilities, for only then can the student see how they manage to cope (often very effectively) with the situation. By talking to the patient in depth they also learn what handicaps they actually face.

Suitable objectives

On independent visits students can learn:

* the effects of an impairment on a patient's life;
* the ways patients overcome disabilities;
* the environmental changes that can reduce the adverse effects of disabilities;
* the attitudes of society to disabled people;
* how structures and actions in society handicap disabled people;
* to recognize their own feelings towards disability;
* to develop a caring attitude towards people with disabilities.

The basic approach to independent visits has already been discussed in Chapter 6. To realize these objectives, students should be encouraged to visit the disabled person on more than one occasion. It is also valuable to talk at length to any other members of the household. If it is possible to accompany the disabled person outside the home, this can increase their understanding of handicaps people face in society at large.

Visiting young patients with cerebral palsy, severe learning difficulties, or muscular dystrophy provides students with many opportunities to learn, not only from the children themselves but also from the parents. Many parents are particularly articulate about the handicaps they and their child have faced. Discussion about how the problem was first recognized and conveyed to the family often gives insights into attitudes in society, including the health care professions. Approaches can also be made through self-help groups whose members are often prepared to talk to students because they feel very strongly about their own past experience.

It is not only visits to patients with severe locomotor conditions or multiple congenital conditions that provides a good learning experience. Patients with chronic airways disease, vascular disease, or eczema can also be severely handicapped. It can be useful for students to see how a common condition, often dismissed as comparatively easy to manage, causes a great deal of distress because of the way that it is viewed in society.

Debriefing after visits is essential. The students may have met a considerable amount of anger or distress and need to be able to share their emotions. Other professionals involved with the care of the disabled person might suitably provide this debriefing.

PRIMARY HEALTH CARE TEAM ATTACHMENTS

The range of people involved in the care of patients with disability means that learning should not be restricted to a medical perspective. Learners need to discover the roles of the different members, to learn to respect the input they provide, and to explore how a team functions to provide a comprehensive and integrated service to the patient. One way to do this is through attachments to primary care team members.

Suitable objectives

Through attachments to members of the primary care team students can learn:

* The principles of teamwork in the care of patients with disability;
* how the roles of team members contribute to the reduction of handicap;
* how the roles of team members are perceived by other members and patients;
* the place of the patient and informal carers within the team.

As students determine their objectives, they should not just learn about the workers but have a chance to see the workers in action and talk to them about their experience. In this field three groups of worker can provide valuable insights: the community district nurse, the physiotherapist, and the social worker. Each has a different relationship to the primary care team. This provides good opportunities for discussing some of the problems of teamwork.

The community/district nurse

Community nurses play a key role in enabling people to function within the community. They are particularly concerned with people whose disabilities confine them to a house (which includes many elderly people). Much of the work of such staff is with the frail elderly and severely disabled at home. This work includes:

* a wide range of technical procedures (e.g. insulin injection, ulcer dressing);
* monitoring health and well-being;
* identifying opportunities for preventing illness;
* identifying opportunities for the use of aids to prevent handicap;
* identifying treatable physical and mental illness;
* co-ordination of the work of members of the nursing team and of other domiciliary services;
* educating and enabling patients and carers.

As nurses, they are not only involved with the direct care of people. More importantly, they facilitate and enable patients and their carers to function more effectively. They provide insights into the way the internal strengths of disabled people are enhanced.

Students need to understand the key role of community nurses in maintaining seriously ill patients in the community, especially as much of their work may be little noticed by doctors. Future hospital doctors need to be aware of the availability of nursing services in the community if they are to plan continuing care, and community attachments may be the only opportunity in their career to learn at first hand about district nursing care. This will be achieved best if time is spent with community nurses exploring, discussing, and reflecting on their work. This should mean an early start as the central role of the community nurse is emphasized by the first visits of the day, which are often for insulin injections. The student should be exposed to a range of community nursing tasks, and understand that for many of these, contact between doctor and nurse may be extremely infrequent: community nurses largely manage their own caseload and make a range of management decisions without any need to refer for medical advice.

The district nurse is usually a core member of the primary care team and will work reasonably closely with a general practitioner, including attendance at formal or informal team meetings. Students should join in these meetings, especially if a disabled patient they have themselves seen is being discussed. They should observe the working of the team meeting and be able to discuss this working with key participants.

After the time spent with the nurse, or at the team meeting, students should be encouraged to reflect on how it has affected their perceptions.

The physiotherapist

Time spent with a physiotherapist in the community provides a different insight into the care of disabled people. The physiotherapist will be able to show how patients can be taught to overcome some disabilities by relearning skills using different muscles. They will also be able to show how certain aids can be used for the same purpose. There will be an emphasis on restoration of function. Physiotherapists are less likely to be attached to the core primary care team and will give different insights into communication between professionals. The care of many severely disabled people is the responsibility of a secondary care team. Many physiotherapists work closely with secondary care staff, but within the community. Again, the physiotherapist will be able to enlighten students on the reasons and the advantages and disadvantages of this.

The social worker

Social workers nowadays seldom work as part of the primary health care team—there are few attached or liaison social workers. On the other hand, the development of community care means community-care managers are responsible for bringing together a wide range of services to maintain disabled people within the community. This is a parallel team to the primary health care team, but one with which there needs to be close links. Contact with a social services department, and particularly with a community-care manager, can develop understanding of the way such links can develop.

PROJECTS

There are many different disabilities but a special study project focusing on a single issue can still be valuable, providing a good exemplar. A number of aspects of long-term disability make this area especially suitable for student projects both of a qualitative and a quantitative nature. These include:

1. *Prevalence*: many disabling conditions have a high prevalence in the community.
2. *Identification*: patients with disabling conditions can be clearly identified from morbidity registers and computer databases.
3. *Accessibility*: these conditions often mean that patients are restricted in employment or mobility, and may therefore be easier to contact at home.
4. *Clearly defined outcomes*: for many conditions it is possible to look for a clear outcome. For instance, level of control of diabetes, peak flow levels in asthma, or mobility levels for musculoskeletal conditions.
5. *Wide variety of resource utilization*: provides considerable scope for student exploration.

These factors mean students can expect to find an interesting and feasible project while they are learning about the needs of disabled people and the handicaps they experience.

Suitable objectives

During project work students can learn:

- the prevalence of a disabling condition;
- the identification of intermediate outcomes in the care of people with disabling conditions;
- the range of resources available to reduce disability and handicap;
- how to audit the use of these resources.

When choosing projects to enhance learning about disability and handicap it is important to ensure that the project is achievable within the time and resources available.

A survey of care

Students can look at the morbidity register on the computer and identify a population of patients with a specific condition (e.g. epilepsy). They can then survey the records of all those patients to ascertain what management is being provided and what evidence there is that the patient's condition is properly controlled (using agreed parameters). They could then visit a number of patients who exhibit both good control and poor control to discuss the patient's perspectives and to identify possible reasons for the lack of control.

A survey of the community

Students could carry out a project on epilepsy in a totally different way. They could look at how patients with epilepsy are viewed in the community. One project might involve discussions with self-help groups and employers. Another might consider how people in a number of different situations would manage a fit. This might involve a survey of the first aid training of policemen, St John's Ambulance volunteers, and people responsible for sports facilities.

LEARNING ABOUT DYING

Whenever disease and illness are considered, the possibility of death is a natural concern. This is particularly so for students. Death is often remote from their personal experience and therefore viewed with much anxiety. Helping students face these anxieties and consider what skills they need is an essential part of medical education. They must learn to deal with people who are dying and with their relatives. They must learn to manage the bereavement.

Unfortunately, there is considerable evidence that this area has received low priority in the past. At times it has been isolated from other parts of the course and given a special status where students are told 'Today you will have your session on giving bad news and death'. Learning about death and bereavement needs to be integrated in such a way that students perceive it as one aspect of working with patients in different stages of the life cycle.

Learning about dying is also an area where working together with other professionals is important. At the time of a patient's death no professional is an 'island, entire of itself'. Nurses and other workers will be involved. It is heartless for doctors to do the bare minimum of care at times of terminal care and death and leave other professionals to take the brunt without considering their emotional needs.

At first sight the care of the dying might be considered an area more appropriate to hospital learning than the community setting. However, although death commonly takes place in institutions, the time leading up to death and the period of bereavement is a community experience. Students must consider the needs in that setting.

ONE-TO-ONE TEACHING

Community-based learning often allows for a close relationship with a community tutor such as a general practitioner. On home visits, especially to a terminally ill patient or a recently bereaved family, there is the real opportunity to talk in depth about some of the emotions that are felt, and to discuss aspects of sensitivity and empathy. One student was totally changed when he saw the tears in the eyes of an older GP as that GP left the death-bed of a patient known for many years. Back in the car the first question was 'So it is alright if a doctor is seen crying then?'

Suitable objectives

In one-to-one sessions students can learn:

- the needs of patients and carers in the final phase of life;
- how to communicate with patients and carers at this time;
- how to recognize, accept, and manage the emotions of the patient and carers;

- how to recognize, accept, and manage one's own emotions and those of other health professionals.

Tutors must not neglect opportunities to discuss these matters with students. Such opportunities are not always obvious. In the example of the tearful GP the situation was clear and so was the emotion being displayed. However, sometimes in a surgery a bereaved person can raise the issue of a death some time previously. The doctor may deal with this *en passant*, aware of a long period of continuing help and counselling. The student may be unaware of this and see the brief comment as dismissive. The tutor may also be unaware that some passing reference to a death is highly charged emotionally for a student. Sensitivity and alertness are required. It should not be assumed that students are able to cope with discussion of these issues in the same way as colleagues might: maybe we should not assume it of those colleagues!

SMALL-GROUP LEARNING

Discussion with a trusted tutor is one safe place to raise issues concerned with death. The small group should be another haven to explore personal ideas, responses, and the many questions that relate to death. This depends on the group members having had the opportunity to get to know and respect each other. In the small group it should be safe to raise the unspeakable questions such as those about euthanasia (which will be discussed further in Chapter 15).

It is also possible to test out those difficult questions of what to say, how much to say and when to say it. The old question of 'To tell or not to tell', can be stripped down to the essential 'How do I feel about telling this patient at this time?'

Suitable objectives

In small groups students can learn to:

- explore and evaluate different approaches to informing patients about death;
- develop their own skills in informing patients and carers;
- explore their own feelings when faced with death and the failure to cure;
- use their own emotional responses positively.

It is easy to avoid these issues, and to use the small group to explore purely clinical management issues, such as pain relief. Although important, they should not distract from the need to evaluate more personal aspects of care. For this reason care needs to be taken on the selection of material for the small-group discussion. It is also important to allow the students to find ways of sharing their own feelings and not being inhibited by the presence of an experienced tutor.

The role-play session

Students should not be faced with a real practical experience of having to inform a patient about impending death or the death of a relative. However, a major fear is that they will be faced with the need to do this soon after qualification without having been properly prepared. In small groups they can role-play both doctors and patients or relatives. A series of roles can be prepared in advance for the students. Two students then perform the roles, and the group discusses what has happened using the rules of feedback discussed in Chapter 14. Larger groups may be divided into trios of 'doctor', 'patient', and 'observer' so that more approaches can be tried out. The trios can share their approaches afterwards to give broader experience. Students must be aware that this is an area where their own personality and value-systems are important. They should avoid the 'falseness' of a taught approach that does not fit in with their own personality. Tutors also need to be alert to the risk that individual students may bring their own real situation (such as a bereavement) into a role-play and suffer as a result.

The clinical problem session

An alternative to role-play is to focus a discussion on a specific clinical problem, preferably one brought by the students themselves (although the tutor may well guide the choice of patient). Suitable problems are those with complex social or ethical issues or situations where communication produced difficulties or conflict. These are preferable to situations where the focus is on the clinical aspects of palliative care.

EXAMPLE 1

One community tutor was working together with a hospital doctor when a patient was admitted following an overdose of illegal drugs. The patient was in his early twenties with a partner and two children. He was comatose and was believed to have been so for 48 hours. There were questions about the likely outcome should the patient recover consciousness. This could be discussed in terms of the possible medical treatments or in terms of the ethics of maintaining life. The tutors opted to focus the discussion on the feelings of the students who were from the same age range and some of whom shared a social background with the patient. In this way it was possible to explore issues that were often less obvious in the case of the death of an older person.

MULTIPROFESSIONAL LEARNING

Death is not managed by doctors alone. Professional colleagues are involved in both mutual action and emotional support. Failure to understand the roles and the experience of such colleagues may mean patients fail to receive the help to which they are entitled. It may also mean that doctors miss out on much needed personal support. One way to prevent this is shared learning with colleagues in other disciplines. This is becoming more common in postgraduate education where there are workshops for primary care teams on subjects as diverse as health promotion and AIDS. The different training backgrounds prior to qualification has made it difficult to organize shared learning at this level in the past. Changes in both medical education and in education of professions allied to medicine may change this. 'Learning WITH' may be more effective than 'learning FROM' a range of disciplines.

Suitable objectives

In multiprofessional learning students can learn to:

- understand how the roles and skills of professional colleagues can be deployed effectively in the care of the terminally ill;
- work together in mutually supportive teams;
- appreciate the emotional needs of team-members and the effects of these.

There are a several different structures for multiprofessional learning. Multiprofessional group seminars can provide a situation where students from different professions can share emotions. However, two approaches might be considered.

1. Multiprofessional input

In this situation the students, who may be from a single profession, have access to a number of different professional resources. In a seminar on death and dying such a group might include doctors, Macmillan nurses, counsellors, and clergy. In a more traditional, form the seminar might consist of a series of presentations by each of the disciplines where their contribution to a specific case is described. There is the danger of the students listening more to the doctors than to the other groups. The seminar may work more effectively if students have been encouraged to consider the issues beforehand and make their own assessment of how the other disciplines might contribute. They can then be encouraged to discuss their ideas with the professionals.

2. The shared experience

This approach can be used when students from a number of professions are attached to the same community setting at the same time. The community nurse may have a field-work student while the GP tutor has a medical student attached. These students can then be involved in one particular case. An opportunity should be provided for them to share their feelings and concerns about that case, preferably with both tutors present. They will often do this informally if the right conditions are in place. Sadly, students from different professions currently get little chance to work together or to take part in joint discussions of this nature.

LEARNING ABOUT THE PRIMARY HEALTH CARE TEAM

The two situations already discussed have shown how working with the primary health care team can help students learn about disability and dying. Previous chapters have considered the role of the team in teaching about the family and health promotion. The primary health care team is clearly involved in achieving several learning objectives. However, there are objectives that focus on the team itself. Future medical care will depend heavily on professional teamwork and students need to learn respect for colleagues and to develop the ability to work in teams. Future leadership roles will depend more on skills than status so, in many instances, leadership will be in the hands of other professionals, especially those with management training. Students need to learn how to be an effective member of an organization and to work with management. This section therefore reviews in more detail how these specific objectives might be achieved. It does this, in particular, by looking again at attachments to practice nurses and then at attachments to administrative staff. Attachments to other team members (such as health visitors, community nurses, physiotherapists, and social workers) have already been discussed and a further example of how such attachments can be used to achieve these objectives is found in Chapter 23.

PRIMARY HEALTH CARE TEAM ATTACHMENTS

The key to promoting a team-centred approach is good experience of attachments with team members.

Suitable objectives

During attachments to other team members students can learn:

- the training and roles of different team members;
- an understanding of the difficulties experienced in team working;
- respect for the skills of the people they are working with;
- skills in communication with different professionals.

In any community attachment it is important that students spend adequate time with all the people who are involved in the work. In a general practice, for instance, they should spend time with all the key workers in the practice, managerial and reception staff, as well as nurses.

Attachments with practice nurses

Practice nurses have developed many new roles over a comparatively short period. Time spent with a practice nurse will help students learn how new nursing skills and perspectives have been introduced. They should be able to explore nurses views about the extended role, and the extent to which they have been instrumental in the changes or responding to changes in demand by patients or doctors. In such discussions, students should learn how other professionals acquire skills from different forms of training. They should also receive insights into the tensions that this produces in teamwork. They need to be encouraged to determine what stereotypes they have and question the validity of these.

During time spent with the practice nurse, the student should understand the increasingly important contribution which practice nurses make to the provision of health care. Students need to see beyond the more traditional reactive modes in which some practice nurses may still operate and have the opportunity to discover their contribution to areas such as health promotion (already discussed in Chapter 12) and chronic disease management. This requires the opportunity to observe the wide range of roles adopted by practice nurses which include:

- Anticipatory care (e.g. new patient checks, advice on immunization).
- Health promotion (e.g. advice on diet, smoking, and relaxation).
- Management of chronic illness (e.g. asthma and hypertension).
- Provision of contraception services.
- Advice on acute minor illness.
- Provision of technical services (e.g. venepuncture).

Time with the practice nurse may also give the student the opportunity to have supervised practice in carrying out a number of practical procedures (e.g. venepuncture, measuring peak flow rate, and giving immunizations).

As with sessions with a doctor, the one-to-one time with a practice nurse requires that time is set aside for discussion and reflection. This may require some alteration of the appointment system.

Attachments with administrative staff

In order to understand and value the role of management and administration in the provision of health care, students need to have some insight into the work of non-clinical staff. Although administrative staff are no less important in hospital settings, it is often easier to explore this in the context of a general practice. A comparatively small organization enables students to relate the work of administrative staff to those clinical staff with whom they also interact.

The student should understand the key roles and responsibilities of the *practice manager* in a general practice team. Among these students should understand how practice managers are involved in:

- *Organization* of surgery and clinic times to meet the needs of the practice population.
- *Co-ordination* of preventive health care programmes for the practice.
- *Management* of human resources (i.e. staff).
- *Interaction* with outside agencies (e.g. health authorities).

In fund-holding practices, time spent with the lead doctor or the *fund manager* will enable the student to learn how a practice with purchasing responsibility balances the need of individual patients against the needs of the whole practice. They will also discover the relationship between a non-medical manager and the clinical staff when it comes to the problems of contracting. They will be able to explore differences in language and approach that affect such a relationship.

Involvement in commissioning, needs assessment and care for defined groups (e.g. child health surveillance) are the areas of work where a practice's responsibilities to its whole registered population is easiest to identify. The practice manager in a non-fundholding practice may still have an input into the commissioning process, particularly through providing information from the practice about the health needs of the practice population. The practice manager may also be able to discuss how the audit programme of a practice is managed.

Time with *reception and clerical staff* can also be used to achieve certain objectives. The roles of administrative and reception staff include:

- First point of contact with patients for requests for appointments, visits, and prescriptions.
- Maintenance of records, (e.g. filing and, sometimes, notes-summarizing).
- Maintenance of registers for preventive health care (e.g. immunisation, cervical cytology, geriatric health checks).

Time spent within reception, even answering the telephone, gives the student insight into the patient's perspective. They can learn why patients feel the need to be seen without delay, or at a particular time of day. They learn the key role of the receptionist in trying to organize patient demand in a way that can be accommodated in surgery times with regular appointments. Perceptions about receptionist are often negative. They can be seen as background workers with only limited skills. Even worse they can be perceived, even by students, as 'dragons at the gate'. Time spent in the reception area, attached to a receptionist, will enable students to overcome such negative views. They will understand the difficulties of people who are now the first contact for patients. They should appreciate the interpersonal skills that are exhibited. They should be able to use their understanding of the behavioural sciences to explore the tensions felt by receptionists and to note how they resolve them. They will also have the opportunity to discuss key attitudinal and ethical issues such as the extent of confidentiality and of patients' rights. As has been reiterated it is important that time is set aside for one-to-one discussion.

MULTIPROFESSIONAL LEARNING

Another approach to developing teamwork is for students to spend time learning together with other professionals. The opportunity to share expectations and values can help students evaluate their own attitudes. It can also improve understanding and skills in communication with colleagues.

As discussed above this approach is still in its infancy in undergraduate training. There are many possibilities of developing it in future, especially as nurses spend more of their training in the community. In the past there has been a problem because colleagues in district nursing and health visiting have not always had time to give to medical students because of their own responsibilities as fieldwork tutors. More shared learning would overcome this difficulty. Patients should not have too many observers at one time, but it is quite possible for people who have observed in different situations to come together for the feedback and discussion.

Suitable objectives

Shared learning will enable students to learn:

- to understand the perceptions, beliefs and expectations of other team members;
- to recognize difficulties in interprofessional communication;
- skills in communicating with other professionals;
- to explore their attitudes to other professions.

Shared learning depends on available facilities. The simplest approach is when professionals from different backgrounds are being taught within the same general practice. The informal contacts that take place can be formalized with mutual benefit. This may be through considering one or two set topics such as asthma or diabetic clinics, a patient confined to home, or a patient with ulcers. If other professions are not being taught within the practice, then joint seminars between groups of students may need to be arranged at a different level.

LECTURES

Lectures may seem inappropriate for learning in an area so dependent on interpersonal skills. Students do need to discover the skills and attitudes of their colleagues at first hand and that cannot occur in a lecture hall. However, there are some aspects of the working of primary health care teams where a lecture may develop understanding.

Suitable objectives

In a lecture students can learn:

- the structure of primary health care teams;
- the resourcing of primary health care teams;
- an understanding of models that explain team-working.

Students require a conceptual framework for the organization of primary health care. Diagrammatic models can illustrate the structures and show how they have emerged from historical developments, how they are specific to particular cultures, and how they can be used to achieve political objectives. At first sight the structure of British primary health care is incomprehensible. Anyone inventing a primary health care system from first hand would never conceive of such a mixture of single-handed and group practices in premises ranging from health authority-owned premises to back rooms of houses. They would not have had such a range of staff employed variously by practices, by health authorities, and on a voluntary basis. They would not have invented a payment system that includes at least four different financing approaches (salary or basic allowance, capitation, fee for service, and target payments). Students do not need to know all the details, but they need to understand why these complex systems have developed. This will help them to comprehend relationships within services and some of the problems that may ensue. Books are unlikely to provide a comprehensive and contemporary framework. Lectures, especially of an interactive nature, can simplify this structure and give and up to date picture in a rapidly changing scene.

Lectures can also be used to build up a picture of the wide range of community resources that exist. Such a picture will provide students with a background structure and understanding of how these resources can be accessed through the primary care team.

14 Learning how to assess patients

In Chapter 4 objectives related to learning about individuals and to learning how to assess patients were presented. Many of these objectives related to communication. This chapter therefore starts with a consideration of how students can learn to communicate. It then takes a wider look at learning how to assess the needs of individuals.

COMMUNICATION

Communication is an essential medical skill. Students need to learn why it is important and to develop their own personal skills in the field. These are required for the assessment of patients, for negotiation of therapy with patients and their relatives, and in order to work with other professionals, both medical and non-medical, involved in the care of patients.

The community is an ideal setting to learn about communication. In a general practice students can witness a wide variety of communication at first hand including:

- the intense communication of the doctor—patient contact;
- formal and informal communications between team members;
- one end of the delicate communication interface between primary and secondary care;
- the difficulties in recording information and using it at a later date.

Students will have opportunities to practice communication with patients and staff. However, it is not enough to simply allow the students to see and experience these different activities and draw their own conclusions. The experiences need to be analysed, evaluated, and used as practical exemplars to enhance their own skills. Many approaches are suitable, ranging from lectures to a large group to the intensive experience of one-to-one analysis of individual consultations of either tutor or student.

LECTURES

Formal lectures given to large groups are not obvious situations for learning the very personal skills of communication. Even a lecturer who is a highly effective communicator, who can keep an audience engrossed for 30 minutes, may not provide the best role model for the interactive communication of clinical work. However, time and resource factors may necessitate work in large groups for part of the time. Awareness of the objectives that can effectively be achieved in the format will be of great help.

Suitable objectives

Through lectures students can:

- Understand the psychology of interpersonal relationships;
- Evaluate evidence on the effects of communication in clinical settings;
- Discover the range of perceptions and expectations of patients;
- Discover a range of approaches to communication.

Lectures can take many formats. They may be structured didactic presentations, illustrative demonstrations, or interactive sessions. The format used will depend on the key objectives. It is important to ensure that the purpose is clear before deciding on the outline.

The didactic lecture

Students need to be aware of the evidence that communication is important in determining the outcome of medical care. Ley (1988) has brought together the evidence that both patient satisfaction and adherence to medical advice are related to doctor—patient communication. Students who fail to appreciate this may be less inclined to review and improve their own particular skills, whereas many others will feel more comfortable when they realize that there is firm scientific evidence of measurable effects of communication on clinical outcome. Such evidence can be presented in a didactic manner using key research findings as illustrations.

Similarly psychological research on the nature of interpersonal relationships can provide useful background for communication-skills training and increase student awareness of potential barriers. Didactic lectures can be particularly good for presenting the latest research and scientific evidence.

The demonstration

Didactic, structured lectures only have a limited place. More useful are demonstrations that show students the range of approaches to communication and the effects of these. These can take various forms.

Videorecordings can bring home the complexity of communication and demonstrate effective and ineffective methods. The ability to replay and to pause means that specific elements can be highlighted. They are especially effective for showing some of the barriers to communication because they can demonstrate how simple changes in consulting room layout, body language, or other non-verbal aspects can alter the interaction. A video replay can look at the defensive postures and the averted eyes or can cone down on the little gestures and sounds that show that the doctor is listening, or not! Verbal cues and question-framing can also be picked out. Videorecordings can also be used demonstrate techniques and skills that improve interaction. A series of videorecordings can be made of the same patient presenting but with the doctor responding in different ways. This can show how the consultation may develop in varying ways as different approaches are used.

Despite the potential, there are drawbacks to the use of videorecording. Visual input is very important but, in this age of television and virtual reality, watchers can have high expectations of the professionalism of any such input. The technology must be up to expectations. Where the consultation has been done with an actor, it is possible for the students to dismiss the situations as false and unreal. With real patients there is the danger of breaching confidentiality. Guidelines for the use of videorecordings of actual patients are, rightly, becoming increasingly strict. The patient must not only have given informed consent to the taking of the videorecording at the time but have had the opportunity to change their mind after the consultation. They must also be aware of the circumstances in which the recording is going to be used, especially if it were to be shown in a lecture theatre. Detailed guidelines such as those agreed for the use of videorecordings in assessment (Fig. 14.1) should be applied to any similar use.

Another way of providing a demonstration is a *live consultation* in the lecture theatre with an actor as a simulated patient. Simulated patients can be used to highlight barriers to a consultation, as in a videorecording. They can also demonstrate how patients might well have different agendas and different expectations at different stages of a medical story.

EXAMPLE 1

Mrs Feltham might present to her general practitioner full of anxiety with a breast lump. The fear prevents any useful discussion beyond how quickly she can be referred. When she consults the surgeon she wants to know what can be done and what the outcome is likely to be, but at the same time may not take in all the implications. An interview with a breast-care nurse pre-operatively may provide an opportunity to consider much more of the emotion surrounding the situation. An actor playing the patient and a trio of professionals can demonstrate these different agendas effectively in a single lecture demonstration.

The interactive lecture

Lectures are likely to be more effective if there is some level of interaction. Ways of developing active learning in lectures have been considered in Chapter 8. For instance, a lecture on the importance of communication can be started by putting the students into buzz groups and asking them to share together one effective and one ineffective communication that they have encountered in the previous few days. Even if the size of audience makes it impossible to get more than minimal feedback students are already considering issues that the lecturer will later bring out.

In lecture-room situations it is often possible to give the students work to do in small groups. Their responses can then be built back into the lecture topic. A lecture

Guidance

1. Medical procedures involving patients may be recorded on videotape, audiotape, or on film, for the purposes of assessment or training, only where the patient has given free and informed consent. Where the recording involves a consultation between doctor and patient, or any other procedure from which the patient may be identified and the recording of which might cause the patient embarrassment or other distress, doctors are responsible for ensuring the following:

a. The patient understand the purpose for which the recording would be used; who would be allowed to see it, including the names of the people, if known; whether copies of the recording would be made; and how long the recording would be kept.

b. The patient understands that a refusal to consent to recording will not affect the quality of care being offered.

c. The patient is given time to consider a consent form and explanatory material which sets out the necessary information in a way which the patient can understand (translations should be provided where necessary).

d. The consent form is neutrally worded, on order not to imply that consent is expected.

e. Where patients are unable to give consent because they suffer from a mental disability or for any other reason, consent must be sought from a close relative

or carer. In the case of children who lack the understanding to consent on their own behalf, the consent of a parent or guardian must be obtained. The person giving consent must understand the rights set out above and below.

f. The recording must be stopped immediately if the patient requests or if, in the doctor's opinion, the recording is reducing the benefit which the patient might derive from the consultation.

g. The patient is invited after the recording to consider whether to vary or withdraw the consent to the use of the recording.

h. Where, following a recording the patient withdraws or fails to confirm consent, the recording is erased as soon as possible.

i. The recording is used only for the purposes for which the patient's consent has been given.

j. The recording is stored with the security required for all confidential medical records.

k. The recording is erased in accordance with the patient's instructions.

These conditions also apply to copies of a video recording.

2. Where a video recording is, or may be, shown to people other than the health care team immediately responsible for the care of the patient at the place

where the recording is made, the following additional safeguards should be applied:

a. The patient must understand that the recording may be shown to people with no responsibility for the patient's health care.

b. The patient must be offered the opportunity to view the recording, in the form in which it is intended to be shown, before the recording is used, and have the right to withdraw consent to the use of the recording, at that stage.

3. Where it is proposed to make a recording from which the patient cannot be identified, it is sufficient for the doctor to give the patient an oral explanation of the purpose of the proposed recording and to seek the patient's consent, which should be recorded in the patient's notes. No recording should be made contrary to the patient's wishes, and no pressure should be placed upon a patient to give consent. In exceptional circumstances, where no recording of a procedure has been planned but an unexpected development during the procedure makes a recording highly desirable on educational grounds, a recording may be made without consent if the patient's consent cannot be sought (for example because of anaesthesia). In such circumstances, the patient's consent must subsequently be obtained before use is made of the recording.

Fig 14.1 Videorecording of consultations between doctors and patients and of other medical procedures, for training and assessment (from GMC 1995 with permission).

on the difficulties of language may begin by asking groups to consider the meaning of several simple words (fit, stroke, cold, fever, bug, or virus are good starters). It is important to make clear how long students will have for their group work within the lecture, and to have techniques, such as the dimmer switch, for recapturing attention and providing some time for feedback from the groups.

SMALL-GROUP LEARNING

Lecture formats can usefully provide basic input and develop student awareness about communication. They are less effective for developing skills or exploring attitudes. Practical opportunities to develop communication skills and history-taking can be provided in a small-group setting. However, great sensitivity is required by tutors. Ability to communicate is perceived as a key social skill, an important part of self-image. Students can feel very threatened if they feel they have a weakness in this area, and are shown up in front of their peers. Classical teaching ward rounds can be considered as small groups. Many tutors will remember their own anxieties when the consultant says 'Ms X will you now take a history from Mr Y . . .' Such anxiety can be even greater when the scrutiny includes videorecording and playback in front of the group.

Small groups can be used effectively to learn basic skills but this is not the only possible use. They are an ideal format for exploring and developing patient-centred and empathic attitudes that are essential to effective communication. They can also provide a safe environment for exploring personal feelings about painful aspects of medical communication.

Suitable objectives

Through small groups students can:

- explore reasons for ineffective communication;
- broaden understanding of the emotional and cognitive needs of patients;
- explore their own emotional reactions and attitudes to patients in a way that helps them establish effective relationships;
- learn how to provide mutual support and encouragement when faced with difficulties in relationships.

Small groups can use many different methods some of which are particularly relevant to the exploration of attitudes. Some examples follow.

Discussion of videorecorded tapes

Groups can discuss videorecordings of consultations. These may be demonstration tapes which are safe because no one present feels personally involved. It is also possible to use recordings carried out by group members prior to the session. In this case the group members will have had a chance to decide whether they feel it is acceptable and appropriate to bring an issue to a group, so again there is a degree of safety.

Discussion of live consultations

Groups can discuss consultations that members carry out during the group session. Consultations may be with real or standardized patients. It is possible to use a fishbowl technique where student and patient sit at a table in a room and the group sits silently (!) around. Alternatively the consultation can be carried out in a separate room connected by a one-way window or closed-circuit cameras. Many students find this particular format more threatening, but whichever setting is used care is required in the way that feedback is given. It is for this reason that Pendleton and his colleagues (Pendleton *et al.* 1984) proposed rules of feedback in developing consultation skills in general practice vocational training. These were:

1. Briefly clarify matters of fact.
2. The doctor in question goes first.
3. Good points first.
4. Recommendations not criticisms.

Such rules are equally important in undergraduate learning. Too many students still complain of being humiliated during their training. This is an area where their individual strengths need recognition. Students require definite feedback on positive elements which should be reinforced throughout their career. They also need to understand that they are being asked to develop their own strengths and to adapt them to the new situations they face. In the group setting, particular emphasis should be placed on ensuring the group considers good points before making recommendations. All members of the group (including the person who has carried out the consultation) can be very keen to say how they would do things better. Although this can be helpful, it can be destructive in retrospect unless the strengths have also been highlighted.

In the feedback rules even the concept of recommendations may be too strong. A useful variant (see Box 1) is to ask students what they might have done differently (if they had not been in a situation of high anxiety). The rest of the group can also say what might have been done differently and to greater effect, but in such a way that a

---

Box 1   Rules for feedback in analysing consultations (modified from Pendleton *et al.* 1984)

1. Clarify factual questions
2. Doctor/student describes what went well and why
3. Rest of group (including patient and tutor) describe what went well and why
4. Doctor/student describes what could have been done differently
5. Rest of group describe what could have been done differently
6. Doctor/student states what they have learnt

student can consider whether that is relevant to their style and approach. If a range of options are proposed by students in discussion, it may be possible to try some of these out with role-play to discover whether they feel comfortable with the proposed option. This approach may extend the range of skills.

Another danger is to get caught up in the technical aspects of the consultation ('Did you ask whether the pain went to the right shoulder?'), and fail to move to communication aspects such as question-framing or feelings.

In using real or standardized patients the focus is likely to be on the basic interactional skills. The final two examples of small group work can build on this but are more relevant to the exploration of attitudes.

The patient—tutor

There are many types of patient simulator. A common practice is to invite volunteers from the general public or from drama schools to learn a standardized role and then perform that role with students. These are the people who can be termed *standardized patients*. They are useful for learning and assessing simple history-taking and basic communication skills. Another approach has been developed: this is to use trained actors with skills in replaying and reflecting on the roles they enter. Such actors have a lay background and this helps them develop insight into the feelings of lay people in different health care situations. They have developed feedback skills which enable them to reflect those feelings to students both while remaining in role and when they come out of their role. This is difficult for real patients who are always emotionally entangled in the situation. Actors working in this way can be seen as both patients and tutors. Such *patient—tutors* can help to bring students face to face with the feelings of patients and help them to reflect on what aspects of their demeanour, attitude, and words engendered such feelings. Both positive and negative feelings should be expressed. It is important that patient—tutors give feedback such as 'I felt it was very easy to talk to you', as it is to tell students 'I wanted to talk about . . . but somehow I felt I couldn't raise the issue'.

Patient—tutors can be used in a wide range of situations. If students want to learn how to motivate people to respond to health-promotion messages they can explore factors that encouraged and hindered such motivation. At the other extreme, patient—tutors can explore with students aspects of giving bad news. Small groups enhance this exploration. When students are encouraged to consider these feelings with their peers they discover a range of responses and can explore alternative approaches.

Student role-play

Patient—tutors are expensive resources. Some of the same objectives can be achieved by allowing students to role-play patients as well as doctors. Students may be provided with a pre-designed scenario or they may develop their own roles based on a patient they have seen in their clinical attachments. The student plays the role of a patient with one of their peers acting as the health professional. Following the consultation the student, who has been playing the patient, can discuss the feelings engendered. Students are usually kind to their peers but it is still possible to bring to the surface feelings of frustration or anxiety as well as feelings of comfort and caring. The experience of these emotions, even in a role-play, is important in the development of empathy.

EXAMPLE 2

One student was very intolerant of smokers. He was asked to play the role of a heavy smoker with chronic bronchitis presenting with an acute exacerbation. His colleague started some health education about smoking. The student concerned was amazed at the anger and irritation that he felt within his role. As the patient he felt he was being attacked when vulnerable. After this episode he felt he had greater empathy with real smokers.

ONE-TO-ONE TEACHING

There is no doubt of the importance of one-to-one teaching in communication. The use of individual feedback following videorecording or audiorecording of actual consultations has been shown to be one of the most effective ways of developing communication skills. This is especially in practical areas, such as the ratio of open to closed questions, the clarification of answers and the use of summarizing. Facilities are easily available in many community settings.

Suitable objectives

Small-group training cannot provide as intensive feedback as the one-to-one situation. On the other hand, one-to-one teaching may not be as effective in attitudinal exploration as there are only a limited number of ideas and values to explore. In one to one teaching, therefore, students can learn how to:

- achieve an effective rapport with patients;
- discover the main reasons for attendance;
- discover their perceptions of health and their reasons for consulation patients (i.e their ideas, concerns, and expectations);
- use silence (and other listening skills) effectively;
- clarify the problems and summarize them;
- inform the patients of the nature of the problem and adapt their information-giving to the patient's needs;
- negotiate a plan;
- end the consultation.

In planning one-to-one teaching on communication, whether it be through the use of direct observation or through the analysis of pre-recorded consultations, one major consideration, already mentioned, must never be forgotten. Communication is a very personal social skill. Students feel vulnerable if they are considered deficient in this area. Those who are weakest and need most help may be the most vulnerable. This was why Pendleton and his colleagues (1984) originally derived their rules of feedback (see Box 1, p.123). They have to be followed more closely in a one-to-one situation with a tutor who may be perceived as an expert. Tutors may offer different approaches but, if this is done, the student should see them as offers not directions: alternative approaches, which work well for a tutor, may not fit the style and personality of the student.

A further way to reduce the threat from this learning method is to start from the learners' own needs. Students know what they find difficult in communication: it may be the patient who 'won't stop talking and let you get on with your history', or 'deaf patients'. Students are often anxious about patients asking difficult questions and finding themselves not knowing what to say, a reflection of their concern about giving bad news which needs to be addressed. There are several ways to deal with these different concerns.

Direct observation of real consultations

This can take place in the consulting room as suggested in Chapter 3, or via closed-circuit television if the setting is suitably wired. The tutor watches the interview. After the history has been taken the student may require some immediate feedback. In the early learning years it would be difficult for students to negotiate management plans with patients and the tutor may take over at this point. In later years the student may consult with the tutor after completing the history and examination, agree an appropriate management plan, and then return to negotiate that plan with the patient. This will help to build the student's confidence. At the end of the consultation the tutor can give feedback on the whole process.

Review of pre-recorded interviews

Another possibility is for the student to record interviews with patients. This may be done in a consulting room or at the patient's home. The tutor is not directly involved at the time of interview and it is less appropriate for the student to carry out an initial assessment or negotiate management. Patients may be chosen because they can help students learn how to explore complex problems, deal with people from different backgrounds, or develop skills in dealing with the talkative or deaf patient. The students may review the interviews themselves before they report back to the tutor. Alternatively, student and tutor can review the recording together using the rules of feedback.

The skills laboratory

A third approach is for students to carry out interviews in special facilities remote from the community setting where their interviews are watched, either directly or on CCTV. These skills laboratories (see Chapter 8) are less likely to provide real-time consultations but they may provide a resource in the form of standardized patients or patient—tutors. This gives the opportunity for students to practice complex informing and negotiating skills without any risk to patients and receive feedback from either a tutor or a patient—tutor.

ASSESSMENT OF THE NEEDS OF AN INDIVIDUAL

Communication is only one aspect of assessing the needs of individual patients. Traditionally, the arts of history-taking and clinical examination go together with appropriate use of investigation in making an overall assessment as the basis for developing a management plan. Working with patients in the community helps students to approach this essential medical task with a much broader vision:

- They learn to take into account the patients background. They should understand the patient as a whole person who has psychological and emotional needs and who lives in a social milieu and a physical environment.
- They learn to consider the patient's own perceptions of the symptoms they are suffering. They realize that a needs-assessment must include the ideas, concerns, and expectations of the patient and of those close to the patient. They realize that the reaction of people to illness has a major effect on the options available.
- They learn that there is a high level of ambiguity and uncertainty surrounding presentations of illness. The classical textbook syndromes appear only rarely and the first manifestations of illness are often through vague symptoms such as tiredness or pain in the stomach. Assessment has to take account of this uncertainty and to recognize the self-limiting (and often undiagnosed) nature of many symptoms.
- They learn the need to make safe assessments that recognize danger but do not subject patients to untoward investigations or anxiety.

ONE-TO-ONE TEACHING

There is no better place to learn the skills associated with assessment than the consulting room. Students can watch the experienced doctor who uses a few well chosen questions, examinations, and investigations to make a definition of the patient's problems. They can perceive how past knowledge of the patient, time, and an understanding of basic epidemiology are all vital components of this assessment. They will have wide opportunities to learn and to practice examination skills and at the same time to consider how to choose an appropriate level of examination.

Suitable objectives

Through one-to-one teaching can learn:

- specific examination skills;
- to assess a patient's mental state;
- to focus their examination;
- to use investigations rationally;

- the use of simple clinical epidemiology;
- the use of time as a diagnostic tool;
- the value of an understanding of past history and of physical and social environment.

To make the best use of the time in the consulting room, it is not enough for students to simply sit and observe. Their time must be structured in some way, whilst allowing full advantage to be taken of the wide range of patients attending. The very variety of presentations and the highly unstructured nature of many presenting problems are themselves part of the learning process. There may need to be two concurrent agendas in any session:

Opportunistic learning of practical skills

Students need every opportunity to practise their examination skills, even simple chest auscultation or sphygmomanometry on normal people. If the patient is willing, the student should be allowed to replicate every examination the tutor does. In the process, the tutor will often note a weakness in the technique which can be corrected. In most cases, community tutors will be able to demonstrate appropriate examination techniques as effectively as their hospital counterparts. For many areas of examination the experience that students would get in a consultant-led clinic is very small. A general practitioner will be able to provide many more opportunities for students to see eardrums, to describe rashes or to examine knees, backs, or eyes. At times, the medical school may offer specific sessions for tutors to learn the techniques that are recommended for students.

Students will, however, comment that GPs are more restrained in their use of examination and often do not carry out a full examination even of a single system. The reasons for this need to be discussed. This means being prepared to defend a decision not to carry out a particular procedure because the likelihood of it producing additional evidence is remote. The evidence for a particular examination should be judged on the same grounds as ordering an investigation.

Structured sessions to focus key points

Although opportunistic learning is important, careful structuring of sessions means that key points are covered. One session might consider the concept of time as a tool. In this session the student is asked to note all the instances where the tutor specifically made use of time as a way of managing a condition. This will include statements such as 'I expect it to be better in three or four days. If not, come back!' It will also include patients who have returned after a period of observation. Another session might focus on the use of investigations, with the aim of showing how many positively aided assessment.

Over a number of sessions students may be asked to keep a logbook. Through this they can collect their own brief experience of the epidemiology of general practice. They can compare such a log book with other surveys or with their hospital experience.

A useful experience for them is to compare the patients who attend a practice with those who attend an A&E department.

INDEPENDENT VISITS

In order to develop patient-centred assessments students need to learn how individuals react to illness. This requires time talking to patients. Patients are often more relaxed and more free to talk within their own homes. For this reason students should be encouraged to carry out independent visits to the homes.

Suitable objectives

Through independent visits students learn:

* the social and environmental background to the patients life and health problems;
* how patients react to an illness;
* how the patient's household and family react to an illness;
* the patient's perceptions of health and feelings about their problems.

In organizing independent visits tutors need to consider logistic and educational factors. Logistic factors include the consent of the patient, the timing, transport, and identification and were discussed in Chapter 5. Educational factors include careful choice of patients and provision of background information.

Visits arranged by general practices

Many patients are happy to entertain students and to invite them into their homes. However, there are times when it is not appropriate to introduce students either because of the trauma that the patient and family are suffering or because there are aspects of their life that patients would rather not reveal. It is important never to assume that patients will be prepared to see students, even if they have consented before. Each visit must be negotiated, preferably by the clinical worker closest in contact. Students should also be encouraged to check an appointment nearer the time, especially if it has been made in advance.

Patients need to be selected to match learning objectives. It is important that patients are reasonably articulate about their background and their perceptions although, occasionally, it will be the carer who is going to be the main informant. There is always gain from spending time with people, especially those who come from a different background or who have had different life experiences. Students gain most when the patients are able to talk freely about these experiences.

Both patients and students need to be prepared. The patient should understand why the student is there or they may not see the relevance of some questions the student asks. Students should discuss with tutors in advance the objectives for the visit and any concerns they may have about how it will be carried out. The visit will be easier if the students are provided with a briefing document. This should include some background about the areas that will be illustrated by meeting this patient and some of the topics that should be covered. For instance, a visit to an elderly housebound patient will be more valuable if the student has prior information on the range of problems that affect such people; the proportion of people of different ages who are totally housebound; their housing circumstances and the services that can be provided for them.

Community follow-up schemes

Hospital doctors may also arrange community visits. This may occur in association with hospital-discharge planning (see Chapter 5). Closely linked to this are community follow-up schemes for students when patients are discharged from hospital. These may be arranged by the students in hospital before the patients leave hospital. These schemes enable students to discover the background of patients, their perceptions of the illness, and in particular to follow a natural history of the condition which is seldom experienced in hospital. They can follow the patient through to the rehabilitation and recovery stages or through a decline and deterioration. Suitable patients for such community follow-up are those recovering from myocardial infarcts or surgery. In these cases, the assessment of their needs includes a realization that they have to readjust to life in the community or to work. There is often a marked difference between the perceptions of patient, carer, and professionals about work capacity.

SMALL-GROUP LEARNING

Students need to learn how decision-making is carried out in medical practice and to assess different aspects of this. They also need to learn to cope with uncertainty and ambiguity. There can be considerable advantages in sharing experiences about these issues with peers in small group sessions.

Suitable objectives

In small groups students learn to:

* identify levels of uncertainty in clinical assessment;
* identify approaches to managing uncertainty;
* identify the wide range of factors in reaching a clinical decision;
* explore their own decision-making skills.

Clinical logic and decision-making are often taught in the context of the history, examination and investigation of an individual patient. The assumption can be made that by a logical inductive process collecting information from these sources leads to a small range of differential diagnoses. These can be quickly elucidated by further investigation leading to a clear cut diagnostic statement. However, consider the presentation of a young woman with a three-day history of a sore throat, some exudate on the tonsils, cervical lymphadenopathy, and a feeling of tiredness. At this stage, investigations can neither confirm nor refute a possible diagnosis of infectious mononucleosis. The student has to learn to cope with the uncertainty. Equally, the effect of that possible diagnosis on the woman (who may be facing exams) and on her boyfriend mean that the final problem-statement will never be the bare diagnosis 'Infectious mononucleosis', but 'Infectious mononucleosis in a final-year student who is currently job-seeking'. General practitioners are aware of these wider connotations and will discuss them in their one-to-one teaching. However, a problem-based small-group session enables students to explore this in a broader way.

Problem-based group sessions

Problem-based learning (PBL) has been discussed in Chapter 2 where it was pointed out that using problems as a basis for learning is not the same as learning problem-solving skills. PBL can, however, be used to broaden students knowledge and understanding of the factors that are involved in an assessment. Students are presented with a simple problem and asked to consider together what they need to learn in order to understand and assess that problem. As in all PBL they will need to go through a number of stages. At the University of Limburg in Maastricht, the Netherlands, this process is called the 'Seven Jump' after a Dutch children's song. The stages are shown in Box 2 and are described by David and Patel (1995). Once the problem is clarified and defined the use of this process will affect consideration of the assessment of the individual in several ways. Reflection on possible explanations (step 3) may provide a broader range of definitions of a problem, increasing the complexity of the situation. The same step may show how the level of uncertainty could be reduced by defining actions or learning goals.

In PBL, the problem has to be carefully designed to trigger appropriate learning objectives. In clinical teaching, such as the subject of this chapter, the problem provided may be very brief. The process can also be adapted. A group can be presented with the statement: 'A 16-year-old girl presents with a two-day history of abdominal pain'. As the group produces possible explanations it is immediately clear that further information is required to elucidate this problem. They can propose a series of questions that might be answered from previous knowledge, history, examination, or investigations. For

---

Box 2 The 'Seven Jump' (from David and Patel 1995)

1. Clarify terms and concepts in the problem which are unknown to you
2. Define the problem (i.e. list the phenomena to be explained)
3. Explain the problem; try to produce as many different explanations for the phenomena as you can think of. Use prior knowledge and common sense
4. Arrange the explanations proposed; try to produce a coherent description of the processes that you think underline the phenomena
5. Formulate learning goals
6. Attempt to fill the gaps in your knowledge through individual study
7. Share your findings with your group and try to integrate the knowledge acquired into a comprehensive explanation for the phenomena. Check whether you know enough

each question they should explain why it will help them. It may also be appropriate for the group to look at the problem in a hypothetico-deductive way, to decide only on the first two or three questions to ask, and to await the answers to those before considering further questions.

One series of questions may relate to how ill the patient was at the moment of presentation: In the example given, was the patient doubled up in pain, or did she walk in quite normally? Students can see how such questions may help to limit the uncertainty as to whether this is an acute surgical emergency. A second series of questions relating to the same problem might concern the likelihood of a reproductive problem such as pregnancy or sexually transmitted diseases (STD). This might provoke consideration of how social background can affect the approaches that are taken and of how to address these questions. This method allows students to generate hypotheses and to explore how these can be tested. A group of six to eight students will produce a wide range of possible responses. As they discuss the reasons for these responses the understanding of the whole group should be enhanced. This in turn will lead to more effective assessments. It will also help students define the degree of uncertainty and to explore with each other ways of coping with this. In this way, the PBL group can extend beyond its strict remit and consider attitudes to doubt.

CONCLUSION

Learning how to assess patients is a complex task. It requires a good base of knowledge, skills in eliciting the history and clinical signs, and suitable attitudes both to people and to issues such as uncertainty. The areas that have been considered in this chapter are only part of the training that should go on in all parts of the medical course. They show how the community can play an important part.

15 Learning about ethics

Many areas already considered, such as the care of the dying in Chapter 13, have raised ethical issues. It is not possible to approach the problems of death without looking at the ethics of choice or of confidentiality. Equally, it is not possible to investigate assessment of population needs without a consideration of resource allocation. Many of the ethical issues students face in institutional settings tend to be of a high-profile nature such as genetic engineering, abortion, and euthanasia. These issues might be termed 'macro-ethics'. In the community, these problems also exist but will be faced less commonly. However, day by day there are other ethical problems. In every consultation there are ethical considerations of respect for autonomy, equity, and beneficence. These might be termed 'micro-ethics'.

EXAMPLE 1

A new patient wants to register in a general practice following the 1990 contract. The GP will earn money by doing a registration examination and giving advice on health care needs. The patient only wants treatment for a wart and is in a hurry. How much pressure and how much informed consent is there in the discussion that follows?

Students can reflect on such daily experiences and thereby sharpen their own ethical awareness and develop attitudes which can then be used when they are faced with more complex issues in institutions. This has to be done without tutors imposing their own ethical views on the students. Direct imposition of views is rare, but there is a danger of indirect imposition as ethical role-modelling on older or more experienced doctors is as much a risk as other types of such modelling. The aim is to ensure that students have begun a process of exploration and constant review of their own ethical attitudes which will continue throughout their career.

In developing an ethical awareness it is useful to have a framework in which such decisions can be discussed. Seedhouse (1988) has produced an ethical grid which looks at core values such as creating and respecting autonomy, serving needs before wants, and respecting people equally, and then surrounded these with concepts that derive from duties, consequences, and external considerations. Gillon (1985) provides a simpler framework that centres on four considerations of beneficence (the doctor's responsibility to do good to patients), non-maleficence (not doing harm to patients), respect for autonomy, and equity or justice. Teachers should have such a framework to help focus discussions in this area.

ONE-TO-ONE TEACHING

The one-to-one tutorial will often include ethical exploration. The rich experience of a surgery or a home visit will bring up ethical issues which students should be encouraged to think through.

Suitable objectives

In the one-to-one tutorial situation students can learn:

- an understanding of the ethical implications of every patient contact;
- an understanding of the importance of involving patients in decisions about their own care;
- an understanding of the resource implications of clinical decisions;
- an awareness of how ethical conflicts are resolved;
- an attitude that one should explore personal value-systems and how they affect care.

Of the rich range of possible examples two must suffice.

EXAMPLE 2: THE REFERRAL

A patient attends with a history of multiple joint pains. This has persisted for several years and the patient admits that the pains are worse when she is tense and worried. Physical examination and investigation and previous referrals on numerous occasions have been negative but psychological examination has suggested that she is depressed. She requests further referral to a rheumatologist for further investigation. The doctor considers such investigation is unlikely to be in the best interest of the patient as it is diverting her mind to her physical symptoms and preventing her from considering her depression. There will also be 'unnecessary' use of rheumatological resources. Should the doctor, respecting the patient's autonomy, give in to the request or should the doctor, wanting to do the best for the patient, try to persuade her to take a different approach? What effect will the doctor's views have on the communication within the consultation?

EXAMPLE 3: THE SORE THROAT

A patient attends with a history of four-days sore throat. On examination the throat is red and there is a pyrexia of 38°C. The surgery is full and the doctor is running late. Should the doctor spend time discussing the evidence for the value of antibiotics in this situation and so allow the patient to take an informed decision whether or not to take them? Alternatively, does the doctor advise simple analgesics (or prescribe an antibiotic) without explanation on the basis that this is the most cost-effective use of the time?

SMALL-GROUP LEARNING

One-to-one settings can show the range of ethical issues that have to be faced but students may feel inhibited about exploring their own views with a tutor, especially if that tutor has clear views of their own. Within small groups students can explore the approaches and their own attitudes more effectively. For instance, a tutor may have personal views about abortion which mean they refer patients who request this to another doctor. The tutor may be quite open that these are personal views and other views are respected, but many students would be inhibited in discussing this issue in depth with the tutor because of differences in age and experience. With their peers they should feel less inhibition and be able to define their own stance.

Suitable objectives

In small groups students can learn:

* to analyse frameworks for exploring ethical issues;
* to use frameworks to explore and test different approaches;
* to understand and tolerate a range of attitudes;
* to evaluate different ethical standards and attitudes;
* skills in communicating about ethical issues.

There are numerous opportunities for small groups to become involved in ethical issues. Indeed, there is a risk of many long and vague discussions which fail to achieve much understanding and even divert time from other objectives. Students need a fair chance to discuss their own views but ethical discussions should be focused.

The session devoted to an ethical issue

There are many ways to trigger a session devoted to ethical issues. A current case in the papers or a recent television programme can be a good starter whether it is a report of a refusal to provide some treatments to smokers or a documentary on the Dutch approach to euthanasia. Students can be asked to think of all the possible factors that might influence such a decision. Alternatively, students can be encouraged to bring their own concerns to a session. They can be asked to think of an issue they have experienced themselves within a recent period. It is not necessary to restrict these to community-based experiences.

The different factors or student experiences can be listed. At this stage, the tutor may provide a very simple framework by showing links between the different factors or problems: some might be related to questions of equitable uses of resources whereas others might relate to the conflict between a doctor's view of what is best and the patient's own desires. An alternative framework might separate problems of decisions for a single person from those that relate to relationships between two or three people and those that relate to society at large.

Students can then work in buzz groups on two or three problems that illustrate points from the framework. This encourages them to talk, but preferably out of earshot of the tutor, thus releasing the inhibitions. At the end, the groups report back, other relevant points might be introduced, and a summary can be produced that develops further a framework for ethical problem-solving such as those described above.

The session where ethical issues appear

More commonly, an ethical issue will arise in a session devoted to other issues. One or more students may be keen to pursue the issue, for instance in a session on communication in terminal care the issue of euthanasia may be raised. Tutors will have to decide how much time to allow for this. They should be guided by the views of the group as a whole, the objectives of the session and the level of concern being shown. With a macro-ethical issue students can easily spend much time discussing at an abstract level. The tutor should keep two aims in mind:

First, to show students their individual responsibility to decide on a approach to such issues: have they developed a personal ethical framework they can use when they have to make practical decisions?

Second, to point out how even these major issues are only one extreme of a range of decisions. Euthanasia can be seen as the ultimate personal choice issue and this can lead to a discussion on how people make informed choices throughout their life?

MULTIPROFESSIONAL LEARNING

Doctors do not act alone when it comes to many ethical issues. Professional colleagues are also concerned whether actions are acceptable. It is often nurses or other professionals who have to carry out decisions. In two well-known court cases of the last two decades (the cases of Drs Arthur and Cox) it was a nurse who reported the events which led to the arrest and trial of the doctor. In these circumstances of shared responsibility, shared learning makes sense. There is still too little experience of it.

Shared learning could provide the opportunity for a much wider range of views to be taken into account. It could also promote the concept that major decisions need to be taken in a multiprofessional way. This does not only apply to issues like turning off a life-support system or stopping feeding. It also applies to decisions such as a suggestion that a patient goes into residential care or that a practice sets aside time and resources for an asthma clinic. Undergraduate students can benefit from the discovery that future colleagues have a wide range of views that may mirror their own.

Suitable objectives

Shared learning can help students to learn:

• the ethics of other professions;
• skills in explaining their own values and ethics;
• respect for a range of values and attitudes.

Shared learning opportunities should constantly arise if students are meeting their peers in other professions. However, many of the discussions in such situations will take place in unstructured situations. Where group work is done the presence of tutors from more than one profession can enhance the experience.

EXAMPLE 4

A question arises in community psychiatry whether a patient should be brought into hospital under a Section. As well as the clinical factors, this raises the ethical issues of compulsory admission. A group of medical students and a group of social work students might meet and discuss this issue with both medical and social work tutors present.

EXAMPLE 5

A patient expresses concern that reception staff have access to their medical records. This raises issues of confidentiality. A group of medical students and a group of health care administration students might meet and discuss this issue with tutors from both fields.

CONCLUSION

In setting out its attitudinal objectives the General Medical Council used words such as 'recognition' and 'awareness'. They also included two abilities: the ability to cope with uncertainty and to change. All the attitudinal objectives relate to a breadth of vision and an openness. This open, liberal approach to acceptance of different value-systems may seem a norm in a multicultural democracy entering the 21st century but this may be superficial. Many students will have had limited exposure to value systems other than those of their own culture and background, and others will have had little opportunity to explore the basis of the values they have absorbed. Some people may retreat into narrow confines, others become almost nihilistic. Either group may reject, in subtle ways, value-systems they do not agree with. This can apply to someone from a strict religious background who cannot accept aspects of individual choice. It equally applies to the liberal humanist who cannot accept the religious basis of many arguments on the sanctity of life. Providing the opportunity for these basic conceptual differences to be brought into the open and thereby to develop not only awareness but understanding and tolerance is part of the difficult art of teaching ethics.

Part Four

Innovative approaches to learning and teaching in general practice

> Room must always be left for flexibility in the curriculum within a medical school, and it is right that there should be differences in emphasis and in outlook between the individual schools. (Sir Brian Windeyer 1966)

In Part IV, different educators present brief accounts of their experiences of developing and evaluating a range of initiatives in undergraduate medical education. The chapters follow a common format of an introduction or background to the innovation, a description of the course, and finally a report of how it was evaluated. Not all these new initiatives have been successful, some have been discontinued or markedly changed in the light of early evaluation, others are still *sub judice*, but they all provide an opportunity for reflection on how to set and achieve objectives in the community.

Most of these innovations were introduced in the first half of the 1990s and can be seen as parallel thinking in several medical schools. These schools have different needs and are at different stages of course development. Other medical schools have been equally innovative and other examples can be found in the booklet on community-based undergraduate teaching produced by the Association for the Study of Medical Education (ASME) (McCrorie *et al.* 1993). The choice in Part IV is intended to show how different types of innovation can be implemented whether in short attachments or over whole years or courses. It also shows how these can relate to either limited community objectives (working with other professionals), broader community objectives (understanding the patient perspective), or even broader course objectives (the attainment of basic clinical skills).

The first innovation considered (Chapter 16 by McGlade), the family attachment at Queen's University, Belfast, has been running for some time and similar schemes have been emulated at other medical schools using general practice as a base. The two succeeding chapters, by Wykurz and Kelly, look at more radical approaches to bringing students into contact with patients and the community from the earliest years of their course. Readers can relate these to family and community objectives discussed in Chapter 4. Chapter 19 by Graham-Jones and Lawrence considers a more integrated approach to learning about community-based disciplines in the clinical years. Again, this is followed by two more radical approaches to the clinical year: the community-based medical firm at

King's College Hospital, London (Collerton and Booton), and the Cambridge community-based course (Oswald). These develop some themes found in Chapter 5. Gill and Adshead (Chapter 22), Biran (Chapter 23), and Dowrick (Chapter 24) describe initiatives to achieve more limited objectives. The examples relate to cultural awareness, interprofessional learning, and mental health. In Chapter 25, Blackie and Campion describe an innovation using a specific learning approach (the concept of projects discussed in Chapter 6), and finally Bradley (Chapter 26) refocuses the emphasis on developing a reflective practitioner (see Chapter 2) in the concept of student-completed records of learning.

16 The family attachment scheme at Queen's University, Belfast

Kieran McGlade

The scheme, which evolved over several years, was originally squeezed into students' spare time and facilitated by volunteer general practitioner tutors. It is essentially about learning how families and individuals perceive, understand, and manage their own health. The scheme arose out of a belief that medical students would benefit from very early and continuing exposure to patients and that there was a need to provide them with experience of how the practice of medicine works in the community. In recent years, formal curriculum time has been wrested from the basic medical science course to provide one tutorial per term with a GP tutor over the first two years of the medical curriculum. Students are still expected to visit patients in their own time. A lecture course entitled 'Lifestyle and health' takes place at the end of second year and draws on the experience the students have from this family attachment course. With the current reconstruction of the medical curriculum at Queen's, as in many other universities, the family attachment scheme is now a key component and will act as a resource to several other curricular themes.

AIMS

There are many possible aims for the family attachment scheme. The student can:

- observe at first hand the processes of family life and health care;
- begin to gain an understanding of human relationships;
- begin to acquire and develop good communication skills;
- appreciate the importance of good communication with both patients and their relatives and with other professionals involved in their care;
- become aware of the organization and provision of health care in the community;
- become aware of the importance of health promotion in the community;
- become aware of the ethical responsibilities involved in patient care;
- begin to understand the interactions between patient, illness, social, and physical environment.

More specific course objectives relating to these broad aims are given to students at the start of the course.

Following an introductory lecture at the university outlining the scheme and describing its aims and objectives, groups of six medical students are allocated to GP tutors from the very first term. Pairs of students are introduced to patients or families by the GP. They then visit 'their family' at least once a term for the two years of the scheme. Selection of patients is left to the discretion of the GP, having regard to the aims and objectives of the course. The patients do not need to have a complex medical problem to awaken interest but it is probably best if there are some sociomedical issues to link together. It is not necessary for the students to speak to the same family member each time. Indeed, it may be educational for them to be able to speak to other family members to get different perspectives.

The GP also gives a tutorial at his or her surgery for all six students once per term. They are not expected to provide two and a half hours of didactic teaching. Rather, they use the time imaginatively, with active learning being the watchword. Each of the three pairs of students will present to the group what they have learned about their family. For this purpose the keeping of a learning diary is encouraged. Students are encouraged to prepare one or two overhead slides to illustrate their talk. Presentation skills are thus promoted and students learn from each other. A discussion will follow in which the tutor can draw out one or two themes. Students may identify several difficulties they are having (e.g. in interviewing technique) and again the group will be encouraged to discuss these and suggest solutions. Part of the tutorial time will be spent looking forward to the next family visit. Tutors, using prior knowledge of the patients, may wish to make suggestions as to fruitful areas of enquiry for students. They will, however, bear in mind that students should be discovering things for themselves. Students should become familiar with health care provision in the community but overemphasis on medical aspects is discouraged and in particular they should not become bogged down with clinical details. The GP can also spend tutorial time discussing an aspect of community care, and may involve a professional colleague such as a nurse, social worker, or pharmacist. A tutor's guide is provided to assist with ideas for further activities, and a meeting of all tutors is organized about once a year to discuss teaching issues.

ASSESSMENT

At the end of the second year and during the 'Lifestyle and health' lecture course students are expected to produce a 4000–5000 word write-up of their experiences in the family attachment scheme. A set of written guidelines are given and students are encouraged to undertake a critical appraisal of their attachment, reflecting on what they have learned rather than merely providing a factual account of their visits.

NEW DEVELOPMENTS FOR THE SCHEME

A study guide or work book has been devised to enable students to make the best use of the learning opportunities which present. A short video has been produced which adopts a 'fly on the wall' approach to illustrate to new students how the scheme works in practice. It follows several first-year students as they visit patients, prepare presentations, and take part in tutorials. The same video can also be used to help in the orientation of new tutors and new patients to the scheme.

Within the new curriculum it is hoped that vertical and horizontal integration will be facilitated by a series of seminars throughout the first two years that will be concerned with such themes as 'disability in the community' and 'employment and health'. Students will be encouraged to draw on their individual and collective experiences of the family attachment scheme to contribute to the discussion.

Finally, it is recognized that this is a continuously evolving course. The new curriculum should help promote the scheme and allow protected time for students to take full advantage of these important learning opportunities.

17 The Community Module:
adopting a community-oriented approach in partnership with the community

Geoff Wykurz

INITIATING A PARTNERSHIP

"Our Community Health Council has long been saying that medical education needs to move out into the community, because doctors do not seem to understand people: they just look on them as slabs in beds. The CHC said to the Colleges that there was another way: bring your students out and we will do something about it. We talked to the Colleges who listened, and after a lot of pressure and discussion the Community Module arrived."

In these words Janet Richardson of the City and Hackney Community Health Council (CHC) sums up the impetus for the introduction of the Community Module and alludes to the way the innovation was introduced (Wykurz 1992). The CHC's ambitions coincided with the emerging alliance between the local medical colleges of the St Bartholomew's and Royal London School of Medicine. Although students entered medical school motivated to meet people, no programmed involvement in the community existed to tap and channel this enthusiasm. Restructuring of the curriculum created the opportunity to introduce a community-based element for first-year students.

Consulting community organizations and public health departments at the outset ensured that the module reflected local health issues. This approach reflects the principles adopted by the World Health Organization for community-based educational programmes that have been valuable reference points during the module's development (WHO 1987).

LEARNING IN PARTNERSHIP

The Community Module adopts an experiential approach to explore a holistic perspective to health and health care in a community context. Nearly 300 students are involved in the module annually and this requires a large number of tutors. Very few tutors are medical. Most are recruited from community organizations representative of the diversity of ethnic communities in East London. They share ownership of the module and can introduce changes to reflect current local issues and concerns.

Opportunities are created for students to learn about a local community, social issues, inequality (in relation to ethnicity, class, gender, sexuality, age, and disability), the delivery of services and access to health care. They are also expected to develop skills in observation and reflection, verbal and written communication, and team-work. Students are particularly encouraged to develop an empathic response to the needs and circumstances of people in the community and an awareness of their responsibilities to the individuals they meet and the communities within which they pursue their studies.

First-year element

During their second term students work in groups of four, within a cluster of twelve and supported by a tutor to focus on a community issue. The majority select an issue from a prescribed list that includes subjects such as housing, mental health, the needs of the elderly, or under-fives. Students are matched to tutors interested in their declared preference.

During a field-work block of two and a half days students meet people who live and/or work locally to gain their perspective on the assigned issue. Tutors recommend people for students to contact (phone cards are provided). Students also prepare a community profile related to their community issue. Each group prepares a poster with a supplementary sheet on the theme of their community issue which they present to students and tutors. Some students pursue the aims of the module by working with patient-partners, and this is described in Chapter 18.

Second-year element

In the fourth term, students choose from over 40 community studies proposed by the community tutors. Eighteen three-hour sessions are allocated which includes a block week to pursue field-work. There are three formats: students may work in pairs on placements (based with a local community organization); in groups of six for projects (focusing on a specific issue); or in patient-partner attachments (linked to individual health service users). Criteria for community studies encourage proposals that elicit the perspectives of local people and engage the students in activities that have potential community benefit. This approach encourages a high degree of motivation and commitment from tutors and students alike. Tutors brief students about tasks associated with their study (e.g. interviewing or use of questionnaires). Students undertaking projects submit protocols to a special sub committee of the District Ethics Committee and guidelines on personal safety and security are provided. Students write individual reports and participate in the preparation of a group product. Each group decides the most appropriate audience with whom to share what they have learnt (e.g. a community group, GPs, or the general public). They then choose the most appropriate format (e.g. a presentation, poster, or leaflet).

PARTNERSHIP IN PRACTICE

The Community Module has become an established element of the curriculum that is the product of sustained commitment, creativity, and energy of tutors. Each year, the community studies offered cover a diverse and stimulating range of relevant topics. In one year, these included: homelessness, the needs of Somali refugees, ophthalmic health, the needs of people with asthma, confidentiality of medical records, coping with death and dying, elderly discharge from hospital, dental care for children with haemophilia, independent accommodation for young people with learning difficulties, and a 'give-up smoking' campaign targeted at Muslim men during Ramadan.

EXAMPLE 1

One community study gave students the task of preparing a leaflet on HIV/AIDS for young people with moderate learning difficulties. Although the project was supervised by a tutor the leaflet was commissioned by the young people for whom the leaflet was intended. Consequently, the students were not only required to research information about HIV/AIDS and the needs of people with learning difficulties, but they were also accountable to a group of young people with a different background to their own. Through the project the students developed a range of communication skills, particularly how to convey a message clearly and accurately to a target audience and the importance of empowering people through information.

EVALUATING THE PARTNERSHIP

Evaluation questionnaires and meetings with students and tutors demonstrates the value of the learning that has taken place and raised several issues discussed below.

Students' perspectives

Students' experiences have generally been positive: they enjoyed meeting 'real people'. For some, their experience has had a major impact, changing their attitudes towards the people they have met with an appreciation of the difficulties they face in maintaining their health, and the health of those they care for, and gaining access to health care. Many develop a holistic perspective as illustrated by the statement of one student who said: 'It will definitely make me see patients as a whole person with a background rather than just a list of symptoms'. This sums up the impact of the experience on their future professional practice. Students also developed an appreciation of the role of voluntary organizations in complementing statutory services and of the importance of health professionals working with them as partners in the task of identifying and responding to health needs. A further positive aspect was the development of a range of communication skills: the confidence to simply chat to people, interview skills, working with health-advocates and interpreters, preparing posters, writing reports, and making presentations to a variety of audiences.

However, not all the students saw the value of the experience: one student took the following view: 'I could spend my time doing other things than communicating with the public. I'm training to be an MD not a social worker'. Some students would prefer more clinically oriented activities and found it difficult to relate their community experience with their other studies. This implied a need for greater integration between the basic sciences, clinical skills, and a community-oriented approach.

Tutors' perspectives

When students are engaged in 'real' work, where there is the potential of having an impact on the lives of people, expectations are high. This can trigger tensions between creating and sustaining stimulating learning experiences for the students and fulfilling the goals of the study in which the tutor has invested considerable time and energy. Tutors valued the opportunity of working with the students and enjoyed their teaching role. Their participation was considered demanding, but worthwhile.

The students' best posters have been displayed in local libraries and most of the community studies generate group products of value to the individuals and organizations that have sponsored them. Leaflets are circulated throughout the area on various issues, reports are prepared that influence the policies of statutory authorities, and presentations are made to professional audiences and community groups that stimulate discussion.

ISSUES

Many issues have arisen:

1. *Student learning.* Students need support to prepare personal learning goals that narrow the depth and breadth of the module's aims for their community study, and need structured support to reflect on their experiences.
2. *Advocacy, translation, and interpretation.* Resources must be maintained to enable students to communicate with people from the diversity of ethnic communities.
3. *Ethics.* Ethical oversight needs to be supportive and not bureaucratic.
4. *Personal safety and travel.* Students need to be alert to issues of safety, but guidelines must not foster a negative attitude towards inner-city areas. Many students express concern about travelling costs.
5. *Integration and timetabling.* Horizontal and vertical integration of a community perspective within the curriculum is necessary and an overloaded timetable can create a negative attitude towards community-based activities.
6. *Assessment.* Assessment needs to consider the process as well as the outcome of learning. Although the diversity of learning opportunities is a strength, achieving consistency in assessment is difficult.
7. *Resourcing tutors.* Tutors bring knowledge, experience, and expertise which must be valued and appropriately remunerated.
8. *Community benefit.* Besides the direct benefits to organizations from the work of students, the module has also been a catalyst for facilitating contact between individuals and agencies to work together on new initiatives.

THE FUTURE

The Community Module is a firmly established part of the curriculum, but is constantly evolving, creating opportunities for further innovation. Examples include:

- promoting a community-oriented approach within other elements of the curriculum;
- establishing an advisory group representative of the local community;
- accrediting and training tutors;
- interprofessional training with nursing students.
- collaborating on community-based research determined by local community groups

Acknowledgements

The Community Module's success is a product of the enthusiasm and commitment of tutors. However, others have given invaluable support, in particular: Roger Feldman, Diana Kelly, Peter McCrorie, and Lesley Rees. The tutor referred to in Example 1 was Barbara Mugeridge of the Stepney Children's Fund, Toynbee Hall.

Financial support from the King's Fund and the Department of Employment's Enterprise in Higher Education programme funded the first two years of the Community Module.

18 Patients as partners in medical education

Diana Kelly

'Patients as Partners' is a learning approach introduced at St. Bartholomew's and the Royal London Hospital School of Medicine. It is based on the belief that the training of doctors needs to be more patient-focused and less disease-oriented. It challenges the traditional passive role of patients in medical education by enabling them to be active facilitators of learning. It also seeks to foster relationships between future doctors and patients based on mutual respect for each other's expertise. Many people feel that they lose their identity and autonomy when they become patients and enter a hospital which is frequently seen as an alien environment and the doctors' domain. It was felt that there was a need to redress the balance to enable students and patients to work together, within a more positive learning relationship.

Supported initially by the King's Fund, Patients as Partners began as a two-year pilot study with a part-time worker. It is an experiential and community-based programme that creates opportunities for students to gain insights into the needs and circumstances of health-service users. A patient-partner is defined as someone who uses the health services. They may be people with a long-term illness or disability, a pregnant woman, or a parent or carer of a child or adult. The programme linked individual students with patient-partners on a one-to-one basis, with students visiting their partners at home and accompanying them on various visits. What makes the programme different from a traditional patient attachment scheme is the status of the patient-partners, who in their role as teachers, support the students in planning their objectives.

The principles and processes adopted by Patients as Partners reflect and reinforce current trends in medical education and the General Medical Council's (1993) recommendations. The principles, which underpin the programme, facilitate a new model of collaborative working between students and patients, which gives recognition to patient-partners as experts, teachers, and assessors with an important influence on medical education.

The patient-partners recruited were representative of the different groups within the East End of London (including the Bengali, Chinese, and Somali communities). Thus, resources were allocated, wherever possible, to meet their particular needs (e.g. interpreting and transport costs). In recognition of their time, skills, and expertise, patient-partners are paid modes remuneration. Safety, security, and ethical guidelines were prepared and discussed with students and patient-partners to ensure that they felt confident in participating in the programme.

Patients as Partners has been introduced as an option within both elements of the Community Module discussed in Chapter 17. This enables the programme to work with students early in their training, within an existing community-oriented framework and in curriculum time. In addition, a small group of first-year clinical students participated in patient-partner attachments in their own time.

All patient-partners are invited to attend meetings in college to discuss what they think medical students should be learning and how they can assist them in the process. Students accompany them to a variety of activities chosen by the patient-partners to enhance their understanding of the factors that affect their health. Visits have included a GP's surgery, out-patient department, and a hospice. Students have also accompanied their patient-partners to a tenants' association meeting to see the links between health and housing and to eat at a pensioners' lunch club, as a direct way of learning about diet and older people.

Students are assessed on their work at the end of the attachment. This takes different forms (e.g. a report or a poster presentation). It is significant that patient-partners assist the tutors with the assessment process, giving the students invaluable insights into their work from the patients' perspective.

EXAMPLE 1

A student was linked with a patient-partner living with AIDS. The patient-partner spent time with the student sharing his considerable knowledge about the illness; he also took her to see his consultant, on a shopping trip, and to his day centre. He encouraged the student to talk with his carer to enable her to learn about his role and how AIDS can affect family and friends. The student noted, in her final report, how her patient-partner had not fitted the stereotype she had expected. She described her learning, not just about HIV and AIDS, but also about issues such as sexuality, medical confidentiality, and the day-to-day reality of coping with a terminal illness.

EXAMPLE 2

Another student worked with a Bengali woman who, as a grandmother, was the carer of various members of her family, including her husband who had a long-term disability caused by a racist attack several years previously. The student was able to meet various members of this extended family and visit two of the family members at their workplaces. The attachment took place during Ramadan so he was encouraged to learn about the importance of this religious festival for Muslims and the reasons for fasting. The student, who had lived in the East End of London for several years, acknowledged his own prior ignorance of the racism in the area and the profound affect this can have on health and well-being.

EXAMPLE 3

The advantages of a long-term attachment can be seen from one student who worked for twelve months with a single mother of three children, one of whom had a chronic lung condition and developmental problems. As well as regular home visits, the patient-partner invited the student to meet the paediatric nurse and to accompany her to her son's school and meet his teacher. The child required daily treatment with an oxygen nebulizer and the patient-partner taught the student how to use the equipment. During the year the family moved accommodation. From living in a damp and overcrowded tower block, the family moved to a small house with a garden – the student saw for herself the links between health and housing in a way which had previously only been academic. As the relationship with her patient-partner developed and sense of trust grew, the student was able to extend her original learning objectives (which focused on the boy's health) to look at the health of the whole family, poverty, and her patient-partner's perspective on compliance with treatment. At the end of the year she reflected on her original assumptions about single parents and the growing respect she now had for her partner bringing up her children alone.

EVALUATION

Students have enjoyed working with patients, and many have reported feeling more confident about talking with patients in the future. The evidence suggests that they have started questioning some of their early assumptions and that their attitudes are evolving to include a respect for health-service users and other health professionals.

Patient—partners have also gained from their experiences. A few reported that their confidence had been enhanced and many have enjoyed making a contribution towards the education of future doctors and are keen to participate in the programme in the future. Several patient—partners felt positive about being able to counter negative stereotypes. One person noted: 'I enjoyed the satisfaction of letting my student see that a lot of elderly people still have the intelligence and ability to lead a full and active life and that we are not all moribund or senile'.

Many people have expressed positive views about the scheme and such comments as those shown in Box 1 demonstrate its potential.

Box 1   Patients as partners: some perspectives

'I am extremely encouraged. My concern is that not enough people are doing Patients as Partners. It is a valuable experience for everyone and needs to be made compulsory'. (Senior consultant)

'After reading my student's report I am hopeful that the medical profession will fully appreciate the importance of bringing students into contact with patients and carers at this early stage in their training'. (Patient-Partner)

'I don't think I will ever forget this experience and I feel that it will help me to relate in a new way to patients'. (First-year medical student)

ISSUES

Many issues have been raised such as:

1. *Integration*. How to integrate Patients as Partners with other aspects of the student's training to embed it within the curriculum.
2. *Optimum time for an attachment*. It should reflect the needs and circumstances of both students and patient-partners.

3. *Assessment*. Posters and reports may not be the most appropriate form of assessment.
4. *Development*: Expansion of the programme at a pace which does not compromise the quality of the process of recruiting, training, and supporting patient-partners.
5. *Resources*: Translation, childcare, and transport are required to enable the full participation of patient-partners.
6. *Accreditation*: How to give formal recognition to patient-partners for their contribution to medical education.

Acknowledgements

I wish to acknowledge the contribution of the patient-partners and students who participated in this new and untried venture, and also the support of Geoff Wykurz.

19 An integrated course in public health and primary care

Susanna Graham-Jones and Martin Lawrence

THE RATIONALE FOR LINKING PUBLIC HEALTH AND PRIMARY CARE

Until recent years, medical students at Oxford University had very little structured teaching in primary care. Each student had two practice attachments of a fortnight each, at the beginning and the end of the three-years clinical course. These were popular, but there was no curriculum as such, and little in the way of staff development for the general practitioners involved. Apart from a single seminar at the end of each attachment, there were no timetabled opportunities for students to reflect with teachers on their very diverse experiences. Similarly, the public health course was run in the traditional manner as a teaching block for 14 to 16 students at a time, covering the fundamentals of epidemiological methods and community medicine. As in most other medical schools, it was difficult to interest medical students, preoccupied with the acquisition of clinical skills, in public health.

When the medical school initiated a review of the curriculum, it invited proposals from its constituent departments. Inspired by changes in other medical schools, which were emphasizing the value of learning opportunities in primary care, a group of members of the joint Department of Public Health and Primary Care proposed an integrated six-week course for students in their second clinical year (the preclinical and clinical courses still being separate). The proposal was in line with guidance from the General Medical Council, which set out to promote experiential learning and reduce formalized, lecture-based teaching in medical schools. More time would be spent in the community, public health issues were to be included and cross-disciplinary integration nurtured.

The argument for the new course was further strengthened by the emerging notion of GPs as purchasers of care (the 'primary care-led NHS'), and by general acceptance of the need for evidence-based medicine. It became clear that doctors of the future would need skills in planning and evaluating health care, both for individuals and for groups of patients. What better way to introduce a new generation of doctors to these public health skills than to demonstrate them in problem-solving exercises applied to real life primary care?

SETTING UP THE NEW COURSE

In the second clinical year, Oxford students rotate through a series of attachments to different core specialties. The community attachment comprises a week of geriatrics, the six-week integrated course in public health and primary care, and a further week in palliative care. Several working parties were set up during a preparatory year to prepare suitable seminars for the new course. The topics chosen were clinical care, communication skills, health promotion, health service organization, uncertainty and decision-making, epidemiology, the patient's perspective, care in the community, and control of disease in the population.

Besides the existing teaching staff, funding was required for two university lecturer posts (part-time) and an administrator. Practice attachments were negotiated by recruiting a further six tutors in general practice as part-time members of the Department, bringing the number of tutor practices up to 20. During the preparatory year, the GP tutors met with members of the Department on a regular monthly basis.

THE COMBINED AGENDA OF THE INTEGRATED COURSE

At the heart of the new course was the idea that students should spend alternate days in the Department and in the practice, developing skills of analysis and critical appraisal under the tutelage of public health professionals, while gaining opportunities to observe and practise consultation skills under the supervision of GP tutors.

Students were encouraged to define their own interests and thus plan their own learning, with GP tutors seen as personal mentors. Each student undertook a family case-study for discussion with the practice team, looking at the social implications of illness, and community care. Whatever the particular clinical interests or skills of students, tutors and students could examine routine decision-making in practice from several different points of view. All decisions involve patients, many might involve the evaluation of relevant evidence from the literature, and many have actual or potential consequences in public health terms.

The Department-based seminars were intended to fuel this focus on clinical decisions and broaden it by taking the wider perspective of public health medicine. Seminars on research methodology, observational studies and trials, critical appraisal, and handling uncertainty provided a scientific basis for clinical practice with individuals and populations. Group projects provided additional opportunities for self-directed learning; having identified a problem themselves, students demonstrated their ability to apply theory to practice-based activities.

Formative assessment was programmed into the course as a nine-station objective structured clinical exercise (OSCE) in the fourth week. This, together with a formal discussion with the GP tutor, provided information about students' strengths and weaknesses. Time was then available to do remedial work under close supervision in the remaining two weeks of the course.

EVALUATION AND FURTHER DEVELOPMENT

Feedback during the first year showed how different the new course felt to the students, conditioned to learning from, indeed imitating, doctors in one specialty at a time. They were beset by culture shock. Student groups varied enormously: some were enthusiastic about the new approach: others seemed overtly resentful of the effort involved. Although they could see the relevance of some of the evidence based approaches in practice, they still struggled with the epidemiological concepts and with traditional public health teaching. The 'integration' messages carefully embedded in the course handbook were often missed or dismissed.

In the second year, we developed a more coherent course outline, with three themes applicable to all fields of medicine: evidence based medicine, patient-centred medicine, and health service delivery. It was important to appoint a co-ordinator for each of the themes. The integrated approach was further developed at a team-building away day, when individual GPs worked for most of the day in pairs or small groups with public health physicians, epidemiologists, or social scientists.

Demonstrations of evidence based learning were incorporated into tutors' meetings, in the hope that such case based learning, using computer based searches and critical reading, would gradually become more popular for tutors and students. The results were positive, with 75% of students declaring in favour of the integrated course, and few expressing frustration at the lack of continuous blocks of time in general practice.

The 'patient-centred care' sessions cover a selection of general practice topics such as consultation skills, ethics, audit, professional stress, chronic disease management and other 'medical' topics. These allow the students the opportunity to practise key skills, and to reflect together on their diverse experiences in practice. Some students value this, while others are extremely anxious for more didactic teaching on the diagnosis and management of clinical topics. GP tutors in Oxford, as in other areas, are being looked to as purveyors of a pre-finals crash course in general medicine, as teaching hospital staff have less and less time for teaching. Under these circumstances, the acquisition of new facts, or even revision, is valued above participative learning by many students.

The Oxford integrated Public Health and Primary Care course reflects the 1990 GMC recommendations for medical education in so far as they can be applied to a six week course in a traditional curriculum. The Department has invested heavily in teaching clinical epidemiology, encouraging students to understand its potential in primary care decision making as part of the popular general practice attachment. Inter-disciplinary collaboration has been, and will remain, an important element in the development of the course.

20 The King's Medical Firm in the Community

Joanna Collerton and Paul Booton

The King's Medical Firm in the Community (KMFC) was the first initiative aiming to teach a major hospital specialty, in this case general medicine, from a primary care base. This chapter describes the background to the firm's inception and its evolution to the present day.

The concept behind KMFC arose from local plans to develop a more community-orientated teaching hospital (the King's 2000 Plan). Medical advances and changes in health service provision were resulting in a fall in in-patient numbers which, together with the increasing specialization of consultants, meant that students attached to traditional hospital medical firms were having less adequate clinical experience. The community offered a more representative case mix, the opportunity to see patients in their psychosocial context, and an experienced group of community-based teachers in the GP tutors who were currently teaching on the general practice firm.

An agreement was reached between the Deans of the Medical School and the Professor of General Practice, to develop an experimental firm in general medicine in local general practices. A lecturer was appointed to lead the project, and undergraduate general practitioner teachers were approached for their views on the desirability and feasibility of such a venture. The GP tutors were enthusiastic and took a major part in the planning of the new firm. From the outset the firm was conceived as a combination of community and hospital experience, and a consultant physician worked alongside the GP tutors to develop and maintain the scheme. The firm, which replaced one of the traditional medical firms that taught first clinical year students, started after two years' planning. The programme has since grown and developed. One-third of the clinical students (approximately 40 a year) are taught on the firm.

The curriculum remains divided into preclinical and clinical periods. The first clinical year comprises an introductory period followed by six firms, each of eight weeks duration. Each group of seven students will undertake two firms in general surgery, one in orthopaedics and rheumatology, one combined firm comprising general practice, psychological medicine, and public health, and two general (internal) medical firms. For a third of the students, one general medical firm will be the KMFC. For students allocated to the firm, KMFC thus comprises 50% of the first clinical year teaching in general (internal) medicine. The KMFC therefore stands beside the other traditional medical firms in the school as an equal, committed to delivering a similar general medical syllabus as each of the other firms. It is organized from the Department of

General Practice by an administrator and a lecturer each employed for four sessions per week. They are supported by a committed group of GP tutors based in South London together with physicians based at King's College Hospital.

Aims

The firm aims to teach general medicine from a combined community and hospital perspective with emphasis on:

1. *Attitudes* to patients as people and to learning as a skill.
2. *Skills* in history-taking, clinical examination, interpretation of investigations, formulation of diagnoses and management plans, together with practical and learning skills.
3. *Knowledge* of common medical problems.

The firm is structured to cover a major system (such as cardiovascular or respiratory systems) each week and teaching is co-ordinated around this theme. This is not intended to prevent a degree of opportunistic teaching that allows students to benefit from the various acute, interesting, or unusual problems that arise. The week begins with a seminar broadly covering the themes of the week, the exact content of which is decided by the students. Three sessions are then spent in general practice with students attached singly to GP tutors or in pairs to larger practices. Here, teaching is based around planned encounters between students and patients concentrating on history-taking and examining skills. Most sessions are GP-led but there is also the opportunity to spend time with other members of the primary health care team such as practice nurses involved in chronic disease management programmes. Learning packs have been developed to encourage students in self-directed learning (Graham and Seabrook 1995). Three sessions are spent at King's College Hospital in ward-based and out-patient teaching led by senior hospital physicians with acute medical experience provided by a weekly attachment to the admitting medical team in casualty. There is also weekly teaching in radiology and therapeutics. The whole of the first clinical year comes together for two sessions per week: for pathology teaching and a new scheme of professional skills workshops.

Student assessment involves a combination of formative and summative elements. At the beginning of the firm, student and tutor complete an assessment form based on the aims of the firm. This is intended to highlight the student's strengths and weaknesses and is used to plan learning during the firm. A similar form is completed midway through the firm to gauge progress and again at the end of the firm when it provides the basis for the tutor's grading of the student. Other end of firm assessments include an 'Objective structured clinical examination' (Harden and Gleeson 1979) and a 'Case presentation project' (based on a patient seen in general practice); results from these, together with the tutor's grade, make up the final grade for the Medical School. Assessment results are discussed with each student individually. The assessment process is mutual and students are also encouraged to comment on tutors' teaching skills.

Tutors are supported by regular tutor meetings and an annual GP tutor weekend which focuses on development of teaching skills. Support is also available from departmental staff and from some of the GP tutors who are designated as 'tutor support person'. Payment was arranged which allows GPs to cut their service provision by 50% for those sessions when students are attached to the practice.

EVALUATION

Evaluation of the firm is considered from three viewpoints: students, who evaluate the firm informally as part of the weekly seminar and more formally by completing a feedback form at the end of the firm; tutors and departmental staff, who review the progress of the firm at bimonthly meetings; and the Medical School, which reviews the firm annually at the Curriculum Review Conference of the Undergraduate Medical Education Committee. The response from students has been positive; they particularly appreciate the organization of the firm, the weekly systems approach, the emphasis on clinical skills, and the one-to-one teaching. Concerns have been raised about the numbers of patients seen; students already used to an overburdened curriculum seem on occasion to prize quantity of patients seen above the quality of the learning experience.

Before the project started, GP tutors were worried that they would not know enough general medicine and that they would not be able to find suitable patients to teach on. Neither of these issues proved a problem and tutors report that they find teaching on KMFC a deeply satisfying experience. The main problem for tutors is finding adequate time to devote to the educational input.

The Medical School has also responded positively, noting in particular that KMFC is more effective in detecting and offering solutions to student problems (both educational and personal) than traditional firms.

Four years on from its inception KMFC continues to develop, and influences medical education at a local and national level. King's College Medical School is developing a new undergraduate curriculum in line with the GMC recommendations and the lessons of the KMFC are being used to develop collaborative hospital and community involvement throughout the new course. The *Widening the horizons in medical education* project (Seabrook *et al.* 1994) used insights gained in developing the KMFC to explore the implications of a substantial move of medical education into the community. Three major initiatives have resulted from that work: an action research project developing groups of practices as student learning centres across South London (which will support a greatly enlarged community-based programme in the new undergraduate curriculum); the teaching potential of Community Trusts is being explored; and 'teaching agreements' between the NHS and community-teaching facilities are being piloted as a way to ensure that community-based teachers receive adequate financial support in return for a high standard of teaching.

21 Developing an experimental parallel-track medical course:
the Cambridge Community-based Clinical Course

Nigel Oswald

REASONS FOR THIS INNOVATION

The main reasons for this innovation were a wish to explore the extent of the unused medical teaching resources outside hospitals and to seek ways of developing co-operative teaching between specialist and generalist teachers in medical education. The innovation is about looking for ways to enhance education and not about coping with the difficulties experienced in traditional courses. The essential elements in this programme are that students are attached as a stable, small group to a single practice for 15 months out of the total clinical course of 27 months. This is intended to enable students to focus on patients' problems, to maintain long-term contact with patients where appropriate, and to develop the skills and attitudes required for effective self-directed learning.

The compartmentalization of curricula, combined with the rapid expansion of medical knowledge, contributes to students' difficulty in understanding the illnesses they see in the context of either the patient's life or problems prevalent in the population. Ways to overcome this have been suggested by the General Medical Council (GMC 1993) and by a number of groups which have advocated exploring the resources offered by medical tutors and patients in the community (Towle 1992). The CCBCC seeks to cut the Gordian knot of compartmentalization by basing students in primary care for a very long attachment which allows them to experience contact with patients in all specialties throughout a considerable length of the course.

IMPLEMENTATION

The ideas for this innovation were conceived in the experience of general practice. They germinated in a year of prolonged study leave working on the history of medicine and followed by part-time study in the history of medical education. Supported by evidence on the current activity of students in teaching hospitals and the potential for teaching in primary care they flowered in an article published in the *Lancet* (Oswald 1989). Putting the proposals into action required the agreement of the Faculty Board of

Clinical Medicine of Cambridge University. This permission was granted through a mixture of positive support and only muted opposition. The Education Committee of the General Medical Council was informed and, after making further enquiries, accepted the proposals subject to regular review by the Committee.

Three main areas remained to be resolved: finance for teaching and accommodation; development of appropriate systems within a general practice; and the recruitment of students. Finance for teaching development was obtained through the allocation of Department of Health-tasked money for general practice and the local decision to devote the resources to this development. Finance for additional teaching accommodation was obtained through the support of the Cambridgeshire Family Health Service Authority. Within the identified practice development of a detailed curriculum for the course was completed, along with a disease index, and a register to help students track patients' referrals to hospital and patients' subsequent hospital contacts. The curriculum was developed by the two clinical teachers in the Cambridge Unit of General Practice. A part-time educationist and a full-time project administrator completed the team. The first student selection was done by publicising the course to all students waiting to join the Cambridge clinical course in the year of implementation. The capacity of the course is four volunteer students per year. Interested students visited the practice and satisfied themselves of the bona fides of the people committed to it. The small number involved and the self-selection preclude any attempt to randomize study and control groups of students.

BRIEF DESCRIPTION OF THE COURSE

Having germinated and flowered, the form in which the course came to fruition has been described in a paper in *Medical Education* (Oswald *et al.* 1995). It began as a feasibility study and feasibility was quickly established. The four students take the same qualifying examination at the same time as their peers, and this places some constraints on the running of the course. Students are not selected for any intention to pursue a career in general practice, and it is important to emphasize that this project is an exercise in educational innovation, not of undergraduate vocational training.

Underlying principles of the course include the idea that most students' clinical experience is derived from the problems of patients of a single general practice and that the students remain in contact with their patients in whatever environment they receive medical care and, where appropriate, for the full length of the attachment. In this way students can obtain teaching from specialists as well as generalists, but always in the context of a patient whose problem can be understood in depth. Students are obliged by the realities of such a course to become highly organized and to make conscious personal choices about their education. This is the basis of effective self-directed learning. Particular emphasis is laid on communication skills, understanding patients' problems in context, and on acknowledging the emotional effects of involvement with patients.

EVALUATION

Preliminary partial evaluations have already been published (Oswald and Jones 1994; Wharton 1995). Each student records their patient contacts on a palm-top computer (Psion 3a). This does not constitute a complete record but permits confidence about the minimum patient contacts and their distribution between specialties and the different elements of the curriculum. This data confirms that the quality and type of clinical experience available to students is appropriate.

Because of the large amount of small-group work undertaken in the course, personal observation and feedback constitute a major part of the evaluation. Clinical skills have been evaluated formally at intervals. The development of communication skills has been observed through videorecording of a hierarchy of tasks using informed patients, simulated patients, and role-play. Formal evaluation of skills in practical procedures have been undertaken, as well as evaluations derived from day-to-day contacts with patients. In a Clinical School with a traditional pass/fail qualifying examination it is gratifying to report that all four students in the first intake passed the first part of their final examination without difficulty. Further and more detailed evaluation will become available as the course develops.

22 Teaching cultural aspects of health

Paramjit S. Gill and David Adshead

BACKGROUND

The United Kingdom is a multiracial, multicultural society, with a large black and ethnic minority population (Balarajan and Soni Raleigh 1992), with variations between different ethnic groups both in health care needs, and in the delivery of services (Hopkins and Bahl 1993; Department of Health 1992). Both doctors and patients experience difficulties when dealing with someone from a different ethnic group (Chugh et al. 1993; Eisenbruch 1989). These difficulties are widely recognized, and have been expressed by junior hospital doctors who felt inadequately trained to assess patients from the different ethnic groups they encountered (Poulton et al. 1986).

Pendleton et al. (1984) have shown that a successful consultation depends on the doctor understanding the patient's health beliefs and norms of behaviour. Further, the General Medical Council (1993) has recommended that medical students should acquire knowledge and understanding of how illness behaviour varies between cultural groups (Objective 1(d)). Such undergraduate teaching about ethnic minority patients as does exist, tends to focus on particular diseases prevalent in certain ethnic minority groups. The broader issues of culture and health are often taught, if at all, by chance rather than by design.

The population of Leeds has a rich ethnic diversity. It was thought that this could be used to help medical students learn about cultural aspects of health. It was found that most medical students in their second preclinical year had not had any previous substantial contact with families from ethnic minority groups. Leeds Medical School had committed itself to preclinical work in communication skills as part of a new curriculum. It was decided to include a module about cultural aspects of health.

CONTENT AND PROCESS

The main objective of the module was that students should become more aware of the importance of cultural factors in health. The students' task in order to achieve this was to find out and report what a doctor would need to bear in mind when dealing with a person from a particular ethnic group. They were then to present their findings in as interesting a fashion as possible. This was to be achieved, as outlined in Fig. 22.1,

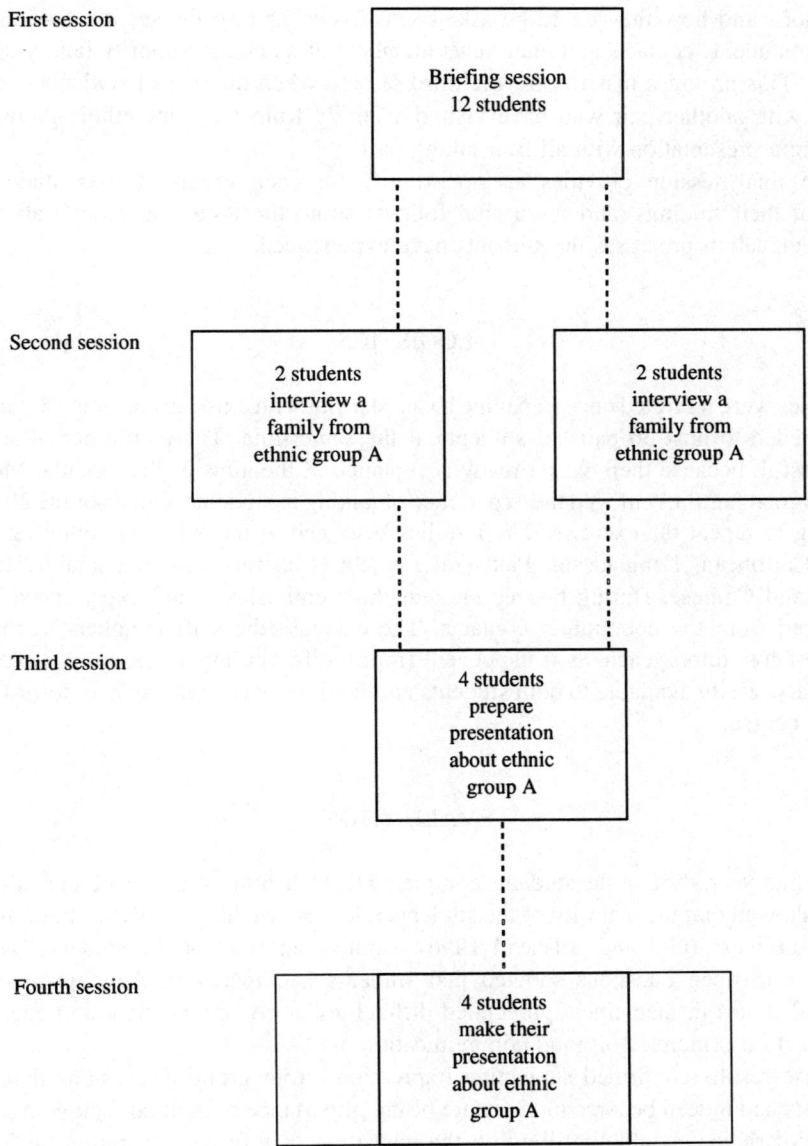

First session

Briefing session
12 students

Second session

2 students
interview a
family from
ethnic group A

2 students
interview a
family from
ethnic group A

Third session

4 students
prepare
presentation
about ethnic
group A

Fourth session

4 students
make their
presentation
about ethnic
group A

Fig. 22.1   Structure of the teaching module for each group of 12 students

with one session a week over four consecutive weeks. The module is run three times a year, on each occasion having five groups of 12 students, thus accommodating 180 students a year.

In the first session, tutors facilitate student discussion in their groups of 12. The students' own ethnic knowledge and role-play are used to determine what are suitable questions and how they could be asked sensitively. During the second session each pair of students contacts and interviews members of an ethnic minority family at their home. This provides material for the third session when the pair of students compare notes with another pair who have visited a family from the same ethnic group, and prepare a presentation with all four taking part.

The final session provides an opportunity for each group of four students to present their findings, and discussion follows about the issues raised and about the communication processes the students have experienced.

LOGISTICS

Families were recruited on a grapevine basis, starting with existing contacts: 30 families are needed to host 30 pairs of students at the same time. The recruitment was very successful, because there was a ready acceptance of the aims of the module. Most of the original families enjoyed the experience of talking to students with 25 of the 30 being willing to repeat the exercise. The families belonged to the following ethnic groups: Afro-Caribbean, Bangladeshi, Pakistani Punjabi (Muslim), Indian Punjabi (Hindu), Sikh, and Chinese. During the recruitment three enthusiastic and experienced tutors emerged from the community contacts. These joined the staff members to make a team of five tutors, each, as it happened, from a different ethnic group. An excellent secretary, easily available to both students and families, was invaluable as co-ordinator of the course.

EVALUATION

In the first year, 89% of the students completed this teaching. Analysis of an evaluation form showed that the majority of the students rated the teaching highly for both interest and usefulness (Gill and Adshead 1996). Content analysis of the students' written answers to open questions showed that students had increased their awareness of cultural issues in medicine, appreciated difficulties of communication, and been able to reflect on principles of good communication.

These results confirmed subjective impressions from group discussions that most students had indeed become more aware of the importance of cultural factors in health. This experience should contribute to the education of a future generation of doctors with more sensitivity and skills in cultural aspects of health.

This is an abridged version of an article that appeared in *Medical Teacher* Vol 18., No 1, 1996.

23 Shadowing other professionals:
a short course introducing preclinical students to other health care professions

Len Biran

Among the objectives proposed by the General Medical Council (1993) (p. 37–39) are an understanding of the importance of communication . . . with other professionals (1 (j)), respect for colleagues (3(a)), and the ability to work effectively as a member of a team (3(h)). At Leeds Medical School a short course was designed to address these objectives. It ran within a communication skills course in the second (preclinical) year of the medical course. As with the course on 'teaching cultural aspects of health' (see Chapter 22), it ran over only four afternoons but evaluation suggested that it had a significant impact on the students.

The course was experiential, rather than didactic, and students were expected to shadow health care professionals, observing their work and discussing it with the professionals themselves, and with their patients. They then had to prepare a report and present it to other students.

PARTICIPATING PROFESSIONS

The health professionals chosen for the shadowing were those that work directly with patients, as it was felt that their work would be the most meaningful to junior medical students.

Of the eligible professions, the following took part:

- hospital and community nurses;
- midwives;
- chiropodists;
- dieticians;
- physiotherapists;
- occupational therapists.

Some of the professionals worked in integrated teams comprising several professions (e.g. teams for care of the elderly or rehabilitation). Where this was the case, several students were attached to the entire team, which took on the responsibility for teaching the whole course, including both the shadowing and the final discussion.

ORGANIZATION

The second-year students were divided into three sections of about 60. For this course students worked in pairs. This meant that about 30 professionals were needed for students to shadow. Eight facilitators were required for the final session. All these tutors were provided by local Health Care Trusts without charge to the medical school (a measure of their support for the aims of the course).

Students received their briefing papers by post, and on the first afternoon dispersed in pairs all over Leeds to meet the designated professional. The students were placed in pairs to stimulate discussion and spent two afternoons with the professional. On the first afternoon, they shadowed the professional and used a structured interview to find out about the less apparent aspects of the profession, such as its responsibilities and training. On the second afternoon, they talked with one or two of the professional's clients, finding out what role the professional played in their lives. The pair spent the third afternoon preparing a report for the final session.

REPORTING BACK

On the final afternoon, students met together in groups of four pairs, each of which had been attached to a different profession. Each pair reported on the profession they shadowed. The educational objectives of this final session were to consolidate the students' knowledge of the profession they shadowed and to widen their knowledge of other professions. A further purpose was to encourage discussion of interprofessional relationships. The facilitators for this session, experienced small-group tutors, were all senior members of non-medical health care professions, most of them of managerial status. Thus, the whole course was taught by non-medical professionals.

The reports presented by the students were structured and contained the following elements:

- Information on the profession: its special skills and in what way its work is similar to or different from a doctor's.
- Information on communication between the profession and doctors: how it collaborates with doctors and whether and how communication could be improved.
- information about the relations between the profession and medical students: what students can learn from the profession and whether and how the relationship between the profession and students could be improved.

EVALUATION

The students' evaluation of the course was very positive. In one sample of 90 students, over four-fifths rated the course highly for interest and usefulness. More detailed analysis showed that most students felt they had learned about the work and importance of the profession they shadowed and a substantial proportion felt they had learned about communicating with patients. Other comments focused on learning about the relationship between the profession and both patients and doctors, and also about teams and team-work.

The professionals who took part in the course were equally supportive. Recruiting and retaining them proved easy. The manager of community nursing service felt that the course raised the morale of community nurses, by showing them that future doctors will be better team members and will appreciate the nurses' role better than present ones. The experience has shown that even a short introduction of medical students to the work of other health care professionals is worthwhile, and that these colleagues are eager to teach and do so skilfully and constructively.

24   Mental health in the community

Chris Dowrick

BACKGROUND

British health care is moving from a hospital focus to a community orientation, and from a doctor-centred approach to one based on collaboration and multidisciplinary teamwork. However, conventional hospital-based medical education and training have failed in the task of enabling new generations of doctors to develop the psychological experience and emotional maturity to cope with the stresses of clinical practice. Some have argued that traditional medical education encouraged the suppression rather than the acknowledgement of feelings (Ross and Stanley 1985), and the search for certainty rather than the acceptance of complexity and ambivalence (Light 1979). These contradictions are acute in the field of mental health. The rapid growth of communications skills-training (Marteau *et al.* 1991) and the creative use of behavioural science courses (de Groot 1987) have gone some way towards redressing these deficiencies, but emotional issues probably still receive less attention in undergraduate medical education than they deserve.

To address this, Liverpool University has run a course entitled 'Mental health in the community'. Before an integrated course was introduced this was run for medical students in the first clinical year. Organized through the Department of Primary Care, it aims to introduce medical students to the wide range of mental health problems that exists in the community, and to the resources available to deal with such problems, including the concept of a network of professional, voluntary, and informal resources with the general practitioner as a gatekeeper. The course also aims to encourage and improve the counselling skills of medical students, and to reduce their anxiety about their own and other people's mental health.

IMPLEMENTATION

The course has been running since a block of curricular time became available in 1986. It was proposed as a co-operative venture between the academic departments of general practice, clinical psychology, and psychiatry, which in itself was a radical initiative at that time. A small co-ordinating group representing each discipline met frequently to discuss out details of structure and content. A critical review of each of the early courses allowed for refinement and adaptation in the light of experience. The original intention was to provide collaborative (shared) teaching sessions but this proved difficult to sustain in practice. After two years, the course was endorsed by the medical faculty as an essential mainstream part of the undergraduate clinical curriculum.

THE COURSE

This lasts for five days and is run three times each year, with 40 to 50 students attending each time. It is composed of a mixture of lectures and presentations and visits to community resources.

Lectures and presentations

The first session provides basic information about the prevalence of mental health problems in the community and discusses the adequacy or otherwise of the resources available to meet these problems. This is followed by a set of small-group discussions on the crucial role of informal social networks in the provision of mental health care, using vignettes based on medical student life. The focus then shifts to primary medical care, with a lecture on the under-diagnosis of psychological problems in general practice, and a discussion of strategies to overcome this. One session is devoted specifically to improving communication and counselling skills. Another covers a variety of topics including family stress and family therapy, death and bereavement, and the political dimension of resource allocation for mental health. On the final morning, a panel of professionals, voluntary workers, and consumers leads a discussion with the students about topics which have interested or dismayed them during the week.

Visits

The three midweek mornings are set aside for visits to relevant organizations and agencies concerned with mental health in the community. A bank of over 50 such venues is now on offer ranging from day-hospitals to group homes, terminal illness hospices to drug rehabilitation centres. Students select in advance their own three visits but are asked to create as much variety for themselves as possible in terms both of setting and of mental health problems. Students also meet a wide range of mental health care workers during these visits, including community psychiatric nurses, social workers, educational psychologists, and voluntary workers in therapeutic communities.

Assessments

Five student teams are each given three hours to prepare a short talk on a topic relevant to the week's work—for instance the disadvantages of community care, the role of the general practitioner in primary care of mental illness, or strategies to prevent 'burnout' in medical personnel. There are also individual assessments by a brief short note paper.

EVALUATION

The course evaluation has been reported in detail elsewhere (Dowrick *et al* 1992). Attendance figures vary, usually following an U-shaped distribution during the week. It is unclear whether such problems with participation reflect student inertia in the face of overwhelming curricular demands, or a set of attitudes and prejudices inherent to this topic. Students consistently rate the community visits as very useful, but are more ambivalent about the teaching sessions! Pre- and post-course questionnaires have also been used to test both knowledge of and attitudes to mental health issues. These have demonstrated 40% improvements in relevant knowledge, in particular knowledge of the prevalence of mental health problems and the range of health care professionals. The attitudinal questionnaire concentrated on anxiety and showed significantly more relaxed attitudes towards mental health problems by the end of the week.

25 Audit projects

Dominic Blackie and Peter Campion

WHY LEARN AUDIT THROUGH PROJECT WORK?

The audit cycle, like the citric acid cycle, is critically important to health and, potentially, just as stupefyingly dull to learn. However, there is one crucial difference: the Krebs' cycle happens whether it is understood or not, unlike the audit cycle, which depends on doctors having the necessary knowledge, skills, and attitudes (Marinker 1990). The almost universal ignorance among clinicians of the details of Krebs' work—despite the time devoted to it in the classical curriculum—is largely irrelevant. On the other hand, the reluctance among clinicians of all disciplines to pursue *rigorous and relevant* clinical audit, despite, for general practitioners, contractual obligation and financial incentives, is arguably detrimental to patient care.

Most individual physicians' lack of meaningful commitment to audit is not principally to do with time, money, or even the manner of its introduction into NHS contracts, but rather because they are not convinced that the effort involved is of practical value to patients. Thus, the central challenge in teaching audit is to communicate the clinical value and the intellectual excitement.

Both can be easily swamped by the tedium of data collection, as any GP or practice nurse in the United Kingdom can testify.

BACKGROUND TO THE LIVERPOOL COURSE

The introduction of clinical audit to UK general practice through the contractual changes of April 1991 has been facilitated by the Family Health Service Authorities (now Health Authorities) via the Medical Audit Advisory Groups (MAAGs). MAAGs are independent bodies, tasked with promoting medical audit in general practice. The Liverpool MAAG, one of four pilot projects, developed a 'practice-centred' model with professional facilitators, in contrast to others which became more centrist (Campion *et al.* 1992). The concept of using part of the audit cycle as the subject of student project work arose from the conjunction of this new audit initiative and a pre-existing general practice project week: students in small groups working on a range of brief practice-based projects, many in the form of patient satisfaction surveys.

The key innovation was to involve general practitioners in the process, by inviting them to submit audit project outlines as bids. A form was sent to all practices in the selected Health Authority area, seeking information about the broad area of general practice to be audited, the specific audit questions to be asked, any standards that might be applied, what methods might be used, and general information about the practice. Members of the Department selected the best ten or twelve projects, using the criteria of educational value and practical relevance. Then the students allocated themselves in groups of four or five to each one.

EDUCATIONAL OBJECTIVES OF AUDIT WEEK

By the end of the week, students should:

(1) understand the concepts of medical audit and appreciate its fundamental importance to clinicians;
(2) be able to devise and carry out a small clinical audit project;
(3) appreciate the effect of working in a team;
(4) have gained some insight into:
    (a) the organization of general practice,
    (b) some of the operational difficulties,
    (c) existing standards of care,
    (d) patient's views of their care.
(5) Have a deeper understanding of the specific topic audited;
(6) Have improved their written and oral presentation skills.

KEY FEATURES OF THE COURSE

Practices bid for the right to participate, which creates a competitive atmosphere between practices, and motivates the practices to invest time in preparation. Students choose their own co-workers and projects. This allows students to develop team-working skills, and to recognize ownership of their project. Each group has a supervisor from among the Departmental staff, to help the group establish a realistic and useful project at the start of the week, and also to interpret the data and advise how best to present it at the end of the course. The majority of the week is timetabled by the students, as would be expected in a project-based course. Help with computing is available from the lecturer in medical informatics, who is a member of staff. There is a detailed course handbook which includes the theoretical basis of audit, and practical guidance on the projects. Finally, for every course the Health Authority involved sponsor monetary prizes, awarded to the groups achieving the most points in a rating exercise involving both staff and students. Travel expenses have been met by the Health Authority or MAAGs, most students using cars to reach the practices, usually attending for two or three days midweek.

In recent years, a wide range of projects has been carried out. In the management area data have been collected on patient satisfaction with appointment systems. Clinically, students have looked at appropriate investigations in people being treated with thyroxine, diabetic care, hormone replacement therapy (and reasons for lack of uptake), and patients' understanding of epilepsy among many others.

On the final day of the course (usually a Friday), the ten groups divide into two sections, and present their projects in two parallel sessions, in which the best two from each are chosen (by student votes). These four then go forward to a final presentation, attended by as many GPs and health authority representatives as possible. Again, the winners are selected by a process of student voting, but with staff and guests also taking part.

COURSE EVALUATION

At the end of each course, students complete a feedback form containing structured rating scales for each component, together with space for free text comments. Over recent years these have shown very high ratings for the attachment to practices, and moderately high for the introductory lectures. In the time available students can only see part of the audit cycle but the course still appears successful because:

1. Students direct their own learning.
2. The projects are directly relevant to patients.
3. Not only do the students learn the basics of audit, but they enjoy the week.
4. Health Authorities acknowledge the importance of the process for practices as well as students.

26 Student-completed records of learning

Colin Bradley

The idea of students completing a contemporaneous record of their clinical experience is certainly not new. The idea of a so-called 'log diary' is a common feature of many undergraduate and postgraduate courses in medical disciplines. However, not all such documents are the same nor, indeed, do they even share a common purpose or set of purposes. Often, they fail to exploit the greatest potential of a student completed record of experience which is to act as a stimulus to reflection on experience that is central to the whole concept of experiential learning and is claimed to be particularly important in the development of professionals (Boud 1985; Schön 1987).

A new type of student completed record has been piloted with students on their final year general practice attachment at the University of Birmingham. The objectives of this new learning tool are that students:

- through its use, should come to appreciate the central significance of the doctor-patient encounter in the delivery of effective primary medical care;
- should be able to perceive the underlying structure of consultations;
- should have had some experience of seeing patients on their own and have reflected on that experience in the light of the course objectives.

For tutors the record is designed to provide insights into the students existing knowledge and understanding. It was also intended that the new record would clarify for tutors and students those course objectives regarded as the most important by the department.

IMPLEMENTATION

The record consists of several sections covering such topics as problem-solving, management of clinical presentations, continuing care of chronic disease, and breaking bad news. Each section consists of:

Preamble: this introduces the concepts relating to the relevant topic (such as the nature of chronic illness as seen in general practice) and possibly a question to check on the student's understanding of the information given. This section also contains suggestions for further reading. *Observation*: in which the student is asked to report in detail on some of their observations of their tutor at work in the area of interest. *Report*: in which the student is asked to describe their own experience of contact with patients selected by the student to illustrate the topic. *Reflection*: in which students detail how they think their experience illustrates the concepts alluded to in the Preamble.

Students have been asked to discuss the content of this document with their GP tutors and GP tutors have been asked to set aside tutorial time with students singly or collectively for this purpose. It should be noted that the philosophy of this new learning tool has much in common with the idea of portfolio-based learning (RCGP 1993) and, indeed, it could form part of such a portfolio. The GP tutor is, in this instance, being used as a type of mentor. The tool, therefore, may help inculcate in students both the ethos and a methodology for lifelong self-directed learning.

Box 1 provides an example of the record of experience.

EVALUATION

The student-completed record has been evaluated by means of questionnaires to GP tutors and to students. Tutors are divided on whether or not it helps them gauge students' existing knowledge. There is more general agreement that the record helps clarify objectives and the priority accorded to different objectives. Almost all agree that it is a positive development. Student evaluations have been similarly encouraging with the great majority claiming to understand its purpose and saying it is easy to complete. Most find it helps them identify and understand course objectives. Free text comments made by students on evaluation forms, while mostly positive, have sometimes contained acerbic criticisms mainly about the amount of work involved.

The development of this new method has not been without its difficulties. Completing it does require a substantial input of time and effort by both students and tutors: an effort that seemed to many to be disproportionate for what is a relatively short (four weeks) clinical attachment. Sometimes, the required clinical experience to allow the conceptual learning and reflection did not occur or was not perceived by student or tutor to have occurred. This was particularly the case with the section on breaking bad news. Students and tutors still seem to struggle with the emphasis placed on conceptual, as opposed to factual, learning emphasized by the document. It required considerable efforts to brief both students and tutors. These efforts were still not ultimately successful in all instances. Finally, it has proven very difficult to find a suitable name for the document.

In its favour, this new learning tool did appear to help make course objectives more explicit and helped both students and tutors prioritize learning goals. It has clearly stimulated some reflection on their experience by students which, after all, was its most fundamental objective.

The evaluation results show the difficulty of applying this in a short attachment. With major curricular revision taking place a common format is being developed for a 'reflective learning tool' to be completed by students in all modules of the new course. This new record will incorporate many of the same features but with rather more emphasis on the reflective elements and less on the information giving.

Box 1   Example of a section of a record of experience for completion by the student

Section Two: Problem Management

The objectives of this section are that students:

- should know what is meant by the biopsychosocial model of illness and how this is applied to the management of patients' problems;
- should appreciate the importance of involving patients in their own management and have had an opportunity to try doing this;
- should be able to formulate reasonable management plans for patients seen by them and have had some experience of trying to negotiate these plans with patients.

Preamble

You will have learnt that the problems presented by patients in general practice can be considered in their physical, psychological, and social dimensions (the so-called 'biopsychosocial model'). Just as the problems have these aspects so too should their management (i.e. there should, ideally, be an attempt to manage the three facets of the patient's problem). Thus, a patient presenting with a sore throat and a temperature may need a prescription for some aspirin gargles to deal with the physical symptoms; some reassurance that it is not a throat cancer to deal with his worry that it might have been one; and a sick note to relieve him of his social obligations until recovery. In addition, the management proposed for the problem(s) should be checked with patients to ensure that it is understood by them; feasible for them to carry out; and acceptable to them. In particular, regarding drug management (the most frequently deployed management strategy) the nature of the problem, the nature of the treatment, its anticipated benefits, and any possible likely adverse effects should all be discussed in terms that are clear and comprehensible to the patient. Likewise, arrangements for further follow-up of the patient's problem should be clear and agreed with the patient.

Observation

Describe an example of your GP tutor applying this biopsychosocial model in the care of patients.

Did you observe your GP tutor considering a variety of possible management options with the patient?

Give details of the options considered and how the patient was involved in the choice of management plan.

Report

Have you had the opportunity to propose management options for patients you have seen on your own?

Were you allowed/encouraged to discuss these with the patient? Describe the process.

Reflection

For the patient seen by your GP tutor, how was the patient's view obtained?

How was the patient's understanding checked?

How useful is it to doctors to obtain patients' views on the management of their clinical problems?

What did the doctor do that facilitated the patient's expression of their views?

Are their any disadvantages to seeking patients' view on their management?

For the patient(s) seen on your own, what management options did you consider?

Can you think of any more options now that you might have considered?

How did you feel about discussing your thoughts about management with the patient?

Part Five
Assessment and testing

> Examinations are formidable even to the best prepared, for the greatest fool may ask more than the wisest man can answer.
>
> (Charles Colton 1780–1832, *Lacon*: I.322)

Education should be enjoyable. Education should be a personal ambition: adult learners will constantly want to develop their knowledge and skills and redefine their attitudes. However, at the end of the day, it is important to know how successful the education has been. This is particularly true in medicine where the public must have confidence that the doctor has the necessary understanding and abilities to diagnose and manage the problems that are presented. The General Medical Council is not only concerned with the curriculum; it is also concerned with assessments. In the United Kingdom, unlike some other countries, there is no national examination to qualify and register doctors. The GMC must be certain that the different medical schools are assessing their students adequately and they therefore monitor the examinations.

Students also need to have some idea of how well they are progressing. They know that at some stage they are going to have to be assessed to make sure they have achieved the necessary competencies (this is termed a *summative assessment*). However, failure at this final stage can be very disheartening. Students need help as they progress in order to be aware of their achievements and limitations. Feedback at this time can help them reassess their learning needs and overcome any weak spots. Tests provided for this purpose are termed *formative assessments*. Closely allied to this are tests that look at potential.

Tutors also need to know whether all the effort that is put into education is effective. The assessment of students is one way of showing this, but it is also important to receive feedback on the educational process and not just the outcome. This is *evaluation of teaching*. It is becoming increasingly important especially as universities are facing teaching assessment exercises organized through the Higher Education Funding Council for England or its equivalents in other parts of the United Kingdom. These will complement the Research Assessment Exercise and will be likely to affect the funds available in future.

Assessments required for the purposes of the public, the student, and the tutor may need to be carried out in different ways. In Part V, Gareth Holsgrove and Lesley Southgate address some of the issues that surround assessment. First, the purposes of assessing medical students are considered in more detail and some of the principles of effective assessment are reviewed. Then in Chapter

29 and 30 there is a detailed consideration of methods of testing knowledge and clinical skills. Communication skills are of such importance that these are considered separately in Chapter 31, and Chapter 32 provides some overall guidelines on assessing clinical competence. Finally, Chapter 33 looks at the question of evaluating the teachers and the course.

These chapters are not confined to discussion of assessment in the community or even assessment of community-based objectives. They provide a much broader canvas. They will enable tutors in the community to consider what assessment techniques are appropriate for both formative and summative purposes in their own field but there are further considerations. As medical education moves into the community, tutors will have an increasing role in the whole assessment procedure. This will be especially true in integrated courses. These chapters should help tutors take an active part in planning and carrying out appropriate assessments.

27 The purpose of assessing medical students

Gareth Holsgrove

Students may be assessed for three different reasons, to measure their potential, their progress, or their attainment. As already mentioned, formative assessment is used to inform students and their teachers about areas of strength and weakness as they progress through the course, while summative assessment counts towards their final mark or grade.

Traditionally, assessment throughout the educational system has placed strong, sometimes overpowering, influence on summative assessment of attainment, with comparatively little attention to monitoring progress and virtually none at all to assessing potential. Where consideration is given to a student's potential, for example, during the selection process for entry to a course, it is usually on the presumption that previous performance indicates aptitude and predicts future performance. In other words, the results of earlier tests of attainment are used as indicators of potential. Although aptitude tests need not differ significantly from tests of achievement, except in their application and interpretation, the latter are often used without much evidence that the interpretation is correct. Attainment tests also tend to be used for monitoring progress. There is certainly some justification in this, but there are other very effective ways of assessing progress which may be overlooked because of the preoccupation with using attainment tests. This chapter will outline some approaches to all three forms of assessment, with a particular emphasis on their role in undergraduate medical education.

ASSESSING POTENTIAL

Training a doctor is a lengthy, demanding, and expensive process. This is an indication of the high value which society places on both the process and outcome of medical education. It is, therefore, quite extraordinary that the principal criterion for entry to medical school is the result of a particular examination (Advanced A Levels in England and Wales), even though these results have never been demonstrated to correlate well with, and thus predict, either results in final medical examinations or with high achievement in the doctor's subsequent career. Like many aspects of educational research, this is a very difficult topic to investigate, but it does pose serious questions about why the selection process should be so dominated by this single factor

(Goldbeck–Wood 1996). The situation is even worse in some other countries (e.g. Australia), where performance in school-leaving examinations may be the one and only consideration in selection. In basing university admission decisions upon candidates' previous achievements, the assumption is made that this will be the best predictor of performance in their chosen course. This may be reasonable where the chosen course and its examinations closely resemble, or logically follow on from, the A-level curriculum. The position becomes less clear-cut in a subject such as medicine, where candidates are unlikely to have previously studied anything similar. The extrapolation from three or four subjects at A-level to the kind of complex interaction of knowledge, skills, and interpersonal characteristics which medical students have to develop appears to be based more on tradition and optimism than on validity.

Most medical schools recognize this limitation and make some attempt to take account of more than A-level results, whether real or predicted. Interviews are commonly held in which the selection panel may consider information from the candidate's curriculum vitae and assess their performance. There are seldom clearly-defined criteria for either of these extra elements and interview panels in the past have been dominated by academic staff. However, some medical schools, aware of the need for broader criteria, are trying to extend their panels to include representatives of community-based disciplines and even lay people.

Even though universities may not yet do so, a number of other organizations put considerable time and resources into assessing the aptitude of candidates for élite or expensive training. For example, potential officers in the armed services or those being selected for fast-track management training in major companies may undergo an extensive series of aptitude tests and psychological profiling. These tests might, for example, challenge teamwork and leadership skills or seek to identify any serious personality deficiency. (It is, incidentally, quite interesting to note how often an analysis of a candidate's handwriting features in aptitude testing of this kind!)

In the United States a Medical College Admission Test (MCAT) has been used since 1991 by over one hundred institutions (Mitchell *et al.* 1994), although not in isolation. In Australia, Monash University is evaluating a structured interview alongside a psychometric test as predictors of performance in the medical course (Tutton 1993). As medical schools move towards less traditional curricula using more adult learning approaches, the need to select students on criteria other than A-level grades becomes greater. The best way to do this has not yet been established.

ASSESSING ATTAINMENT

In the UK educational system, this is usually summative assessment, which counts towards final results in completing the course, rather than assessment of progress, which is discussed in the next section. Summative assessment may occur at various intervals during a course, or at its end, or both. When it occurs during a course it is often (although erroneously) known as continuous assessment; strictly speaking, it should be called continual, in-course, or in-training assessment. Wherever it occurs it is by far the most common aspect of assessment and has an enormous influence on the behaviour of teachers and students. In fact, assessment of attainment is usually the most powerful factor in the entire curriculum, because it determines the *real* curriculum, the one which the students follow, rather than that which the faculty may intend or believe that they follow!

Students will concentrate on material which they think they will be examined on. They will also learn in a way which enables them to cope with the amount and relevance (or irrelevance) of what they must learn. A curriculum with a high factual content presents students with potential learning difficulties. If they cannot gain a good insight into the relevance of this material, then they will be unable to relate it to other things they have learnt or experienced, nor will they appreciate any importance it might have to their future work as doctors. This means that it will be unlikely that they can adopt the deep learning strategies discussed in Chapter 2, which are known to be the most successful. Instead, they will resort to superficial rote learning, which is hard work, boring, unsatisfying, and easily forgotten. The problems are compounded if the examinations reward rote learning by awarding marks for factual recall but fail to assess the application of these facts. Then, students will usually respond with a familiar three-part pattern:

(1) rote learn;
(2) recall facts in examination;
(3) forget.

In medical assessment, there is a strong focus on high-stakes examinations which test student memory for a vast number of facts. This virtually guarantees adoption of this three-part learning behaviour. This creates a serious mismatch between the intentions and objectives of the faculty and the students' view of the real curriculum. This point is discussed in the next chapter when the subject of *consequential validity* is raised. If students are to learn what their tutors' intend them to learn, then that is what must be assessed. The choice of assessment methods must, therefore, be based on the intended outcomes of courses rather than on traditional practices or the existence of a question bank. Some examples of suitable methods are set out in later sections.

Another aspect of the assessment of attainment is the basis on which students may pass or fail the course. If their success is related to their satisfactory attainment of set of specified objectives, then the assessment is said to be *criterion referenced*. If, on the other hand, their success depends on their performance in comparison to that of all the other candidates, then it becomes a *norm referenced* assessment. A familiar example of a criterion referenced test would be the driving test, where the learner will pass if they satisfy the examiner by meeting a list of criteria for safe and competent driving. Their result would not be affected in any way by the number of other learners who had passed or failed. Norm referenced testing is still used in some medical examinations. Here, only a predetermined number of candidates are allowed to pass and, consequently, it can be argued that a major feature of such an examination is to fail people. Indeed, the number of people it fails can be very high. Supporters of this practice may argue that this is the way in which standards are maintained, though this is not educationally defensible. Other proponents of norm referencing admit to using the examination in order to limit membership to their profession. This could be argued to be a misuse of what is essentially an educational instrument for it amounts to little more than an educational cull. The great majority of educationalists are strongly opposed to norm referencing, and the British Medical Association working party on medical education has stated quite plainly that *'norm referenced marking should not be used'* (BMA 1995).

ASSESSMENT OF PROGRESS

This is often known as 'formative assessment'. Progress can be assessed in precisely the same way as a summative assessment since progress is but attainment at one stage of the course compared to that at another stage. There are two problems, however. The first is that many universities are still very secretive about information from summative assessment. They often have regulations which specifically deny access to precise details of results, even though they are potentially extremely useful to students and their tutors. The second problem is that the profound influence of summative assessment may close tutors' minds to the possibilities of using other techniques to assess progress. These other methods, such as well-prepared log books or records of achievement (discussed by Bradley in Chapter 26), can add substantially to the information about progress through the curriculum available to students and their tutors. Records of this kind can also play a valuable part in summative assessment, because they spread the burden of assessment and also present a better picture of what candidates actually do, in contrast to what they know, or know how to do. At present, the potential for assessment of progress is far from being adequately exploited although there is a clear role for involvement of community-based tutors with their close contacts with a few students. At Sheffield, work has been done together with the tutors on developing profiles for assessment which students complete with their tutor and which are intended as learning opportunities (see Usherwood *et al.* 1991) although they also have a summative purpose.

28 Principles of assessment

Gareth Holsgrove

The major principles of assessment can be summarized under three interrelated headings: *reliability, validity,* and *feasibility*. Although they are very important, they are so frequently ignored that even some experienced examiners may be unfamiliar with them. Each acquires a special meaning in the context of educational assessment so this chapter sets out to describe some of the key points in lay terms.

RELIABILITY

Reliability is concerned with the accuracy with which the assessment is made. Among the things which might affect accuracy is the extent to which different examiners marking the same piece of work would independently award similar marks. This is known as *inter-rater reliability*. It is of no importance in computer-marked examinations (e.g. multiple choice questions, MCQs), but may be a major source of unreliability in essay questions and, notoriously, in *viva voce* examinations and selection interviews.

Another important aspect of reliability is the *internal consistency* of a test. Although mathematically complex, the internal consistency describes how well each individual item in a test correlates with each of the other items. It is expressed as *coefficient α*, which may be better-known as Chronbach's alpha (Chronbach *et al.* 1972). It is based on the principle that items in a test should be concerned with the same broad domain. One example might be aspects of general practice: one would expect a good general practitioner to score well in most of the items, whereas someone with poorer knowledge would perform poorly in most. If performance across the items was reasonably consistent, the test would have good internal consistency. If the test contained a dysfunctional item, one which was badly constructed or sampled an unrelated domain, its internal consistency would be reduced. Analysis would be able to identify the rogue item. Obviously, in an extreme case, if every item tested exactly the same thing, then the internal consistency would be almost absolute, which would give a Chronbach's alpha of very close to 1.0. The test developer should seek to compile a test with a number of items (the more the better, as a general rule) which assess aspects of the same domain but without repeatedly testing exactly the same thing. A Chronbach alpha value of 0.8 or higher is usually regarded as satisfactory.

Aside from its value in ensuring that a test is reasonably reliable, in regard to its internal consistency, and in identifying items which impair its reliability, Chronbach's alpha has another very important, yet frequently unrecognized, function. It is the measure of reliability from which the *standard error of measurement* (*SEM*) of an examination is calculated, using the formula:

$$\text{Standard error of measurement} = \sigma \sqrt{(1 - \alpha)}$$

(where sigma is the standard deviation of the marks and alpha is the value of Chronbach's alpha). The SEM can be used to advise examiners on the accuracy of the examination marks for each candidate. This can be illustrated by regarding any examination as a means whereby examiners seek to establish or measure each candidate's 'real' mark, the exact level of the attribute. This is relatively straightforward in a task where the attribute can be measured directly (e.g. measuring someone's height). It becomes much less precise when measuring a less tangible characteristic such as knowledge or ability. In these instances the exact level or 'real' mark will always remain unknown to the examiners. They have to make as close an approximation to it as possible. Furthermore, all examinations contain sources of unreliability. Some of these, such as inter-rater reliability and internal consistency, may be partially under the control of the examiners. Other factors, such as random error, are uncontrollable. The value of the SEM can vary enormously, but in the author's experience of final medical examinations it tends to be in the range 2–4%.

The SEM provides the examiner with an idea of how likely it is that the mark awarded is an accurate reflection of the candidate's knowledge or ability and the confidence with which a judgement can be made. In statistical terms, the SEM gives the examiner a confidence interval for the accuracy of marks awarded in their examination. One SEM indicates a 67% confidence interval. This means examiners can be 67% confident that a candidate's 'real' mark lies within 1 SEM of the mark the obtained in the examination (or, to put it another way, there is a 33% chance that their 'real' mark is not within even one SEM of the one they were given in the exam). The situation is very critical in high-stakes examinations such as final qualifying examinations. Here a 67% confidence interval would not really be enough: certainly it would probably not stand up too well to legal challenge! Examiners might wish to use a confidence limit of 95%, which is two SEMs. Two SEMs is likely to be at least plus or minus 3%. It could be twice, or even three times, as large. This limit might place in doubt the results of a substantial number of candidates whose mark fell within several percentage points of the 'pass mark' or a 'distinction' mark. Traditionally, examiners have either ignored the prospect that their examination results could be inaccurate, or they have used highly unreliable methods, such as vivas, to re-examine borderline candidates. Quality assurance procedures and issues such as accountability and the prospect of legal challenge will demand a much more professional approach to addressing examination reliability.

VALIDITY

The validity of an examination is also a complex issue, but only two aspects are of real importance in this chapter. The first, *content validity*, is well known but the second, *consequential validity*, has only comparatively recently become recognized as a major factor in educational assessment.

Content validity, as its name implies, is concerned with the content of the assessment. Its important aspects are not only that it *appears* to be assessing the right things (this is often known as 'face validity') but that the assessment *representatively samples the curriculum* and includes all, or most of, the essential components. These principles are often violated in multiple-choice questions and vivas, where examiners may concentrate on relatively trivial points. Candidates who expect to be examined on a host of trivial points will usually (and sensibly) make these the focus of their revision.

This raises again the issue of *consequential validity* which refers to the effect an assessment has on the way in which students work and prepare for it. Whatever the noble intentions of those who plan and deliver the curriculum, the effects which assessment exerts on what the students actually do (i.e. the real curriculum) can be profound, especially if they use strategic processing. If the curriculum aims to encourage good practices in learning and professional competence, then these must be assessed and rewarded. Examiners should be encouraged to look critically at the content of the curriculum, relate this to what the assessment process is actually doing, and take note of the ways in which students are preparing for assessment. In other words, examiners must determine whether they are producing a hidden curriculum. This process is likely to lead to substantial changes in assessment.

FEASIBILITY

In theory, examiners can produce extremely reliable examinations which validly cover almost every aspect of the curriculum. The problem is that to do so would demand enormous resources of time, effort, and materials. Under all, but the most exceptional circumstances, this would not be *feasible*. Consequently, the examiners are obliged to trade-off some points in favour of others. Reliability and validity tend to pull in different directions and both may make demands which affect the feasibility of an assessment method, so the process is something of a balancing act. The collaboration of a specialist in medical education might be helpful here, because there are various means whereby assessment procedures can be developed which retain most of the advantages and overcome many of the disadvantages, yet still remain feasible. This process rests on two main principles. The first is to use a variety of assessment methods including, if at all possible, in-course assessment. The second depends on a knowledge of the characteristics of a number of assessment instruments, so that an appropriate test battery can be put together which is acceptably reliable for its purpose. Formative assessment need not be as reliable as summative, whereas high-stakes examinations must be particularly reliable. It must also make an adequate assessment of the curriculum objectives, but not make excessive demands upon people (including the candidates) and resources.

29 Assessing knowledge

Gareth Holsgrove

A recurrent theme in this section has been that the style and outcome of summative assessment is a major determinant of students' learning behaviour. This is especially true in medical education, which is traditionally highly competitive both in student selection and in the many examinations that the students will take, especially if the assessment is norm-referenced. Assessors should be concerned to know the students' achievements in relation to agreed criteria, the curriculum objectives, and, in particular, whether they satisfy the criteria for safe and competent practise. The rank order of their marks is of little interest, particularly when the confidence intervals determined by measures of the reliability of the examination prove that the rank order may be unreliable anyway.

STANDARD SETTING

Having agreed the purpose of a test, a standard should be set. In effect, a standard is the answer to the question: 'How much is enough?' (Livingston and Zieky 1982). It separates those who pass from those who fail, and it will vary according to whether the assessment is one of potential, progress, or achievement. Traditionally, however, for all the talk about maintaining standards, the process of determining what the standards are has been an extraordinarily lax affair. It has relied heavily on experience or 'gut feeling'. The common principal of having a pass mark of 50% is, in most cases, quite dubious. Since there is virtually no attempt to ensure that examinations are of comparable content or difficulty, there is no reason why the pass mark should remain constant.

There are two different kinds of standards, absolute and relative. Both feature in medical education: relative standards in the norm-referenced testing, where there is a comparison between candidates; and absolute standards, independent of the relative performance of different candidates, expressed in terms of what is required in terms of knowledge, skills, or other professional attributes. The counter-educational issues associated with relative standards render them inappropriate for further consideration here. Instead, the two principal methods for setting absolute standards will be briefly described, based on the description of Bowmer *et al.* (1994). Both methods concentrate on identifying the performance of 'borderline' candidates.

Angoff's method

This method requires the group of examiners to begin by discussing their perceived characteristics of a borderline candidate. Based on this discussion, the examiners are asked to independently estimate the number of borderline candidates whom they would expect to answer each question correctly. Obviously, the harder the question, the smaller this proportion would be and in an item such as multiple choice question (MCQ) or a true false question (TFQ), where guessing was a possibility, the smallest proportion should be at least as large as the chance of making a correct guess. These initial, independent, estimates are followed by an item-by-item discussion led by the examiners who gave the largest and smallest estimates for each. Every participant is then given the opportunity to revise their original estimate before the proportions are averaged for each item. They are then totalled across all the items to reach the pass mark for the whole paper.

Ebel's method

This method requires consideration to be given to the relevance as well as the difficulty of each item. This is of particular value in examination development and, were it routinely applied, would help to improve the quality of examination questions by exposing trivial items and identifying any under-representation of essential ones. The method begins in the same way as Angoff's, with a discussion about borderline candidates. However, the process then moves onto a different course with the examiners sorting out the items into a two dimensional grid where *relevance* (essential, important, acceptable, questionable) is plotted against *difficulty* (hard, moderate, easy) for every item. Thus, there are 12 categories available within which, for example, one item may be classified as important and easy, another as questionable and moderate, and so on. When all the items have been categorized in this way, the examiners each make an initial estimate of the number of items in each category that they would expect borderline candidates to answer correctly. As with Angoff's method, this stage is followed by a discussion led by the examiners making the highest and lowest estimates, during which any of the examiners are free to change their minds. When all 12 categories have been discussed, the proportions of correct responses forecast for borderline candidates are averaged in each category, multiplied by the number of items in each category, and finally totalled over all 12 categories to give the pass mark.

TECHNIQUES FOR ASSESSING KNOWLEDGE

Since there are a great many things which doctors need to know, the major preoccupation in medical examinations has been testing knowledge. Although it is increasingly likely that future doctors will need highly developed skills in retrieving information from books and electronic media, rather than attempt to carry it all about in their heads, assessing knowledge is likely to remain an important area in the immediate future. However, examiners are showing much more awareness of the importance of being able to apply knowledge, rather than simply recall it. Therefore, although the assessment of knowledge, clinical skills, communication skills, and competence are covered in separate chapters, there is nowadays a substantial overlap between them and a continuum from the lower cognitive levels of recall to the highest ones of deduction, evaluation, and translation into good clinical practice. There are several well-known methods for testing knowledge, although test developers are continually seeking to improve them or introduce new methods. In particular, there is growing interest in methods which can test the *clinical application* of knowledge. Some traditional and recent methods are reviewed in this chapter.

MULTIPLE CHOICE QUESTIONS AND TRUE/FALSE QUESTIONS

These are generally felt to be the most objective tests and have been around, in broadly similar forms, for almost half a century. Essentially, the format comprises a lead statement, known as the *question stem*, followed by a number of options which are called *branches*. The candidates are required to do one of two things, depending on the type. In the *single correct response* type, they have to identify the one correct option for each item. This, strictly, is the multiple choice question format and normally there are 4 or 5 branches to each question (although other numbers, sometimes as low as 3, have also been used). More common in the United Kingdom, is the format where, for reasons that are historical rather than logical, each question stem is followed by (usually) 5 branches each of which the candidate has to identify as 'true' or 'false'. Strictly speaking, this format should be known as *'true/false questions' (TFQs)*, but in the United Kingdom, they are almost universally known as multiple-choice questions (MCQs). In both MCQs and TFQs, but especially the latter, negative marking may be used. This is a method where a mark is deducted for every incorrect answer in the fanciful belief that this prevents candidates from guessing. When multiple true/false questions are negatively-marked a 'don't know' option is also available. The TFQ format is inherently less reliable than MCQs and this is further jeopardized by the use of negative marking because it introduces a new and uncontrollable variable into the examination, namely each candidate's personal attitude towards venturing an answer to items where they are less than absolutely certain that they are correct. The problems with the multiple true/false format and with negative marking have been well documented elsewhere (e.g. Harden *et al.* 1975; Jolly 1976; Fleming 1988; Wood 1991; Holsgrove 1992, 1994) and there are serious flaws with both the structure and the marking of these items. Unfortunately, many examiners have either remained unaware of these flaws or have chosen (or been obliged) to ignore them. A notable exception to this criticism at the postgraduate level are the examiners for the Membership of the Royal College of General Practitioners (MRCGP), who have discontinued negative marking and are introducing modern alternatives to the multiple true/false format. Both these initatives follow sound educational principles and are proving highly successful.

The principle advantage of MCQs and TFQs is that the answer sheets can be scored very quickly and accurately using optical mark reading (OMR) equipment. This makes it feasible to set examinations consisting of many items and taken by large numbers of candidates, yet still have the marks available shortly after the examination. For this reason, when an examination has a number of components the MCQ or TFQ should be taken last so that the examiners can begin marking the other papers sooner. A second advantage is that both MCQs and TFQs have the potential to test a very large amount of knowledge, albeit mainly straightforward factual recall, in a relatively short time. This advantage can be squandered by examiners who focus on trivia or present candidates with questions that are convoluted, ambiguous, or incomprehensible. A third advantage is that an MCQ examination can be made very reliable, so that pass/fail decisions can be taken with considerable confidence. As has been pointed out, this is less true for TFQs. The US National Board of Medical Examiners' examination discussed on p.190 is an outstanding example of the high reliability of MCQs, with a Chronbach alpha consistently around 0.95.

Unfortunately, many MCQs and most TFQs are of a lamentably poor standard. To a certain extent this is due to one supposed advantage of the method (i.e. that they are easy to write). This did not feature in the list of advantages because it is not true. In fact it is difficult to write good MCQs and very difficult to write TFQs. It is easy to write bad MCQs and TFQs, which partially explains why there are so many around. There are a number of suggestions which can be made for improving MCQs and TFQs, capitalizing on their advantages and overcoming some of their disadvantages:

Construction

1. *Multiple choice questions (MCQs)*:

- All branches for an individual MCQ should be homologous (e.g. all antibiotics, all diagnoses, all anatomical structures, etc).
- If appropriate, branch options should be in a logical order (e.g. if they are numerical they must be in ascending or descending order).
- In MCQs it is very difficult to write one answer which is indisputably the 'most correct' together with 3 or 4 equally plausible distracters. However, as long as *one* is indisputably correct, the others need not be equally-plausible 'wrong' answers.
- Avoid branches such as 'all of the above' and 'none of the above'.

2. *True/false questions (TFQs)*

- In the TFQ format, every item *must* be indisputably true or false. Consequently, multiple true/false items are much more difficult to write because of the problems associated with writing plausible false items.
- Question stems must be clear and unambiguous. Words to avoid include 'usually', 'often', 'is associated with', 'useful', 'may', 'can', and 'good'.
- It is important to avoid negatives, particularly in the question stem where they may lead to double-negatives. On the rare occasions where a negative is necessary in the question stem (such as: 'the following drugs must not be given with xxx') each branch must be phrased positively.

3. *Both MCQs and TFQs*:

- Each branch must follow logically and grammatically from the question stem.

- Include as much of the item as possible in the stem, so the stems should be long and the branches short. In well-written items it should usually be possible to give an answer without looking at the branch options.
- All branches should be of similar length.
- Trick questions must not be used (the purpose of the examination is not to find out whether the candidates can work out what the examiner had in mind when the question was written).
- Absolute terms such as 'always' and 'never' should be avoided (because they are usually false) except, perhaps, in genetics questions.

Content

- Avoid just testing factual recall (it encourages rote learning and is wasteful of testing time because it yields so little information). Instead, concentrate on testing higher-order skills such as interpretation and problem-solving.
- Focus on important concepts, do not waste time and effort on questions about trivial facts.

ALTERNATIVES TO MCQS AND TFQs

There are two options open to examiners who wish to improve their examinations. The first is to dispense with this type of examination altogether, the other is to use an alternative multiple-choice format. In dispensing with MCQs and TFQs the examiner will lose what is probably the only real advantage of the method, its ability to test a large number of candidates with a large number of items. Fortunately, however, there is now an alternative which overcomes many of the disadvantages of the traditional format while retaining the important advantage. Indeed, it also features some additional advantages. This format is known as *extended matching*.

The extended matching format was developed in the United States by Susan Case and David Swanson, of the National Board of Medical Examiners (Case and Swanson 1992). It develops the principle that the majority of the information should be in the question stem, not in the branches, by extending the stem into a clinical vignette. This is accompanied by a list of options, the number of which may vary from about ten to several hundred.

Candidates are required to read the clinical vignette and then select the responses, which can vary in number from question to question, from the list. The answers can be marked on the question paper or entered on a separate sheet. In either case, they can be machine-marked if appropriate equipment is available. Box 1 provides a simple example of two extended-matching items on the theme of chest pain. In this case the question stems are very short, but stems can be used which are much more detailed.

The advantages of this method are clear. They require higher levels of learning than mere factual recall because the candidates must evaluate the information and then make clinical deductions in order to select their responses from the lists of options. Furthermore, even if there were justification for negative marking, it would be unnecessary here because the list of options can be long enough to render the

---

Box 1 An Extended Matching Question (from Case and Swanson 1992)

Chest pain

(a) angina, stable

(b) angina, unstable

(c) aortic dissection

(d) aortic stenosis

(e) herpes zoster

(f) lung cancer

(g) pericarditis

(h) pneumonia

(i) pneumothorax

(j) pulmonary embolus

(k) rib fracture

(l) tuberculosis

For each patient with chest pain, select the most likely diagnosis (each option may be used once, more than once, or not at all)

1. An 18-year-old athlete has a sudden onset of right-sided pleuritic pain, shortness of breath, and decreased breathing sounds on the right.

2. A 52-year-old man has recurrent, achy chest discomfort with exercise; symptoms are relieved by rest.

---

possibility of making a correct blind guess a very remote one. Although the example in Box 1 shows the same list of options being used with more than one clinical scenario, it is also possible to use the same vignette with more than one list of options. For example, the first question might ask which provisional diagnosis was suggested by the vignette and be accompanied by a list of diagnoses. The second could ask which (say, three) laboratory investigations (from a second list of options) should be undertaken immediately, while a third could ask about immediate treatment options from another list.

Another significant advantage is that extended matching items are much easier to write than MCQs because they are clinically based and can be constructed around real cases or typical clinical pictures. In the author's experience, they are most easily written by examiners working together in small groups, with draft items being exchanged with other groups for comments. Furthermore, with thoughtful writing, clinical vignettes can be written for students throughout their medical education from their entry to the preclinical course right through to college examinations.

ESSAYS AND ALTERNATIVES

Long essays

Long essays have been a method of assessment for centuries. Indeed, until recently they were the main or only assessment method used in many courses. Yet they have so many disadvantages in relation to their advantages that they have an ever-diminishing place in education today. They can take several hours to write, although in a formal examination the candidate would probably be allowed an hour at the most, and are very time-consuming to mark. Their advantages are usually held to be that they allow candidates the opportunity to demonstrate that they can assemble thoughts and information in a logical way and present a well-argued case. However, by restricting the time they have in which to do this, the quality of their work is likely to be suboptimal. Sometimes, examiners overcome this problem by giving the essay titles in advance of the examination, so that candidates can prepare a more thorough response. Alternatively, they may set a supervised open-book examination in which candidates can bring relevant textbooks into the examination room and refer to them during their work. This is certainly likely to improve the quality without giving anyone an unfair advantage, but is very rarely allowed in medical examinations even though in their day-to-day work doctors might consult reference books quite often and, therefore, an open-book examination would have an extra element of validity.

Long essays, open-book examinations, articles, and critiques are all time-consuming to mark. Another problem is the high probability that different markers would award different marks to the same piece of work (in other words, the examination may have poor inter-rater reliability). Some examiners, aware of these issues, tend to mark on a very restricted range, for example between 35% and 65% instead of zero to 100%. This conceals the differences between examiners and also makes the examination less discriminating between good and poor candidates. Since this is supposed to be one of the principal functions of most examinations, then using long essays for summative assessment could be regarded as a time-consuming way of achieving comparatively little.

A further disadvantage of long essays is that assessment methods of this type, in marked contrast to MCQs and TFQs, take a long time to sample just a small area of knowledge. This has an adverse effect on both reliability and validity; the former because reliability improves as the number of items increases, the latter because the curriculum is unlikely to be sampled representatively. The validity problem is often made worse because examiners allow candidates a choice over which essay titles they tackle. This breaks a fundamental rule of examinations, that every candidate should do the same examination, hands an unfair advantage to good (or lucky) question spotters and gives the candidates license to miss out chunks of the curriculum in the hope of compensating by getting good marks in other areas. Therefore, these methods may have poor consequential validity because they encourage poor learning and preparation strategies.

Short-answer questions (SAQs)

As the traditional long essay becomes increasingly less feasible, its place is rapidly being taken by short-answer questions. In these, candidates are presented with a number of topics (though, unfortunately, they are still often allowed to choose which they will answer). They usually have about 10 or 15 minutes to spend on each, during which time they may be asked to outline the principal points and, perhaps, show their relationship to each other or to a clinical issue. The examination usually consists of 10 SAQs, although this number can vary substantially. The smaller the number the less reliable the examination will be, so 10 SAQs is probably the smallest number which will prove acceptably reliable for summative assessment. Indeed, it would be better to increase the number of questions and decrease the time available for each, rather than reduce the number below 10.

Reliability is further improved by having a marking schedule which outlines to the examiners exactly what marks should be awarded for. It is essential, however, that all the examiners abide by this schedule, even though they might not completely agree with it. Usually, in an examination consisting of 10 SAQs there are 10 marks available for each and it is essential to emphasize that marks can be awarded right across the range available for each question. Examiners are sometimes heard to argue that: 'I will never give the maximum mark, because that is for perfection and nobody can achieve that'. This assumption is incorrect and can sometimes become a serious problem that penalizes the very best candidates. It serves to illustrate why the marking schedule must show precisely how the marks are to be awarded and why all the examiners must adhere to it. The methods of standard setting outlined earlier can be developed to include reaching a consensus about the marking schedules.

Modified essay questions (MEQs) or patient management problems (PMPs)

These are somewhat similar to SAQs, except that they usually follow different steps in a clinical scenario where the candidate is invited to make short-answer responses to specific issues which arise as the scenario is developed. They have been used in a number of medical examinations including medical finals and the MRCGP. Typically, they begin by presenting the start of a clinical vignette as shown in Box 2. The candidate would write their response on the answer sheet and turn to the next page of the scenario. This would build on the picture and ask a further question. After replying, the candidate would turn to the next step, and so on.

These items are relatively easy to write, although it is important to avoid too many red herrings. Unless the candidates are to hand in each response before gaining access to the next stage of the scenario, it is important not to give answers in later stages so that the earlier responses can be written or altered accordingly. Nevertheless, within these constraints, MEQs are potentially valid and reliable tests of knowledge and its clinical application. It is likely to be a method which will become more commonly used, particularly since it is highly suitable for computer-based assessments.

Box 2   A Modified Essay Question (Three Steps)

1. Mrs A, a 57-year old supermarket checkout operator, visits your surgery for the first time. She complains of [symptoms] Identify five specific questions you would ask during your history-taking.

2. You decide to carry out a physical examination. Identify, with a brief explanation, what you would examine.

3. On examining Mrs A's [system] you found [findings]. Suggest two provisional diagnoses.

One question that arises is the extent to which MEQs could be used to assess students' ability to think in biopsychosocial terms. In the example given in Box 2 appropriate responses to question 1 might relate to psychological and social aspects of the history. The stem of question 3 might be altered to discover whether students could make appropriate triple (triaxial) diagnoses in clinical, individual, and contextual terms. Work has been done on this in the MRCGP examination but there is little experience at present at the undergraduate level.

30 Assessing clinical skills

Gareth Holsgrove

It is not really how much a doctor knows that is so important, it is the effectiveness with which knowledge can be retrieved, organized, combined with technical and interpersonal skills, and used in practice. Consequently, examiners are becoming increasingly interested in methods of assessing these clinical skills. For test-developers, this is a particularly interesting and rewarding area because it presents the challenge of producing assessment methods that must have a high validity, yet need to be acceptably reliable and not excessively demanding of resources. Unlike the recall or application of knowledge, the higher-order skills covered in this and the next two sections (communication skills and competence) cannot be assessed by written tests. They must be observed.

There are three principal ways in which clinical skills can be assessed: observation of actual performance, observation of long and short cases, and the objective structured clinical examination.

OBSERVATION OF ACTUAL PERFORMANCE

The most realistic approach, naturally, is to observe and assess the real thing; in other words, to appraise clinical skills on the basis of day-to-day work. This would certainly have a place in formative assessment and as a component of in-training summative assessment. In either case, some defined criteria are useful, although additional comments from the assessor should also be encouraged. This method has a lesser place in undergraduate education where the students are not yet involved in real life work. However, it can be used to assess performance of certain basic clinical skills which students are regularly asked to perform, such as venepuncture. Observation of actual performance directly or through the use of videotapes is increasingly used at a postgraduate level, especially for skills in communication (discussed in Chapter 31).

CLINICAL ASSESSMENTS: LONG AND SHORT CASES

In a formal examination, which would usually, although not invariably, be a summative assessment, it would be necessary to exercise more control over the situation in order to make the best use of available resources and ensure adequate coverage of the range of clinical skills. Three methods have a place here. The two most common are the long and short cases, in which a real patient is examined and the candidate questioned about their findings.

In the *long case*, which may take between 30 minutes and an hour, the candidate is likely to use a considerable range of skills (communication, diagnostic, etc.) but, extraordinarily, in many long-case examinations they are not observed using them at all. After students have left the patient, they may simply be questioned about what they did and what they found by examiners who were not present during the procedures. This is a waste of an excellent opportunity. The argument for examiners to observe long cases is a very strong one. There is also a need for the observation and questioning to be carried out using a set of appropriate criteria.

Short cases typically consist of students being asked to carry out a series of examinations over a period of about 15 minutes. They are normally observed throughout by one or more examiners, so better use is made of time and resources. However, only a limited number of skills can be tested in the time available, thus limiting the reliability. As in the assessment of routine clinical work or long cases, short cases can yield better information if the examiners base their observations on defined criteria and have also been properly briefed.

OBJECTIVE STRUCTURED CLINICAL EXAMINATIONS (OSCE)

The fourth method of assessing clinical skills was first introduced over 20 years ago as a means of avoiding some of the disadvantages of the traditional clinical examination (Harden *et al.* 1975). Described variously as the objective structured examination and the structured clinical examination, it is now almost universally known as the OSCE (objective structured clinical examination). However, despite its long pedigree, the use of OSCEs for summative assessment is still surprisingly limited, though it is used more frequently for formative assessment.

The OSCE is one of a number of types of multi-station clinical examination (MUSCLEs) (Bingham *et al.* 1994) in which candidates are confronted with a series of clinical tasks. These may include such topics as taking a clinical history, taking a blood sample from a model arm, preparing an injection, suturing, and interpreting radiological images or pathology reports. Typically, candidates will spend five minutes at each station moving from one to the next at the timekeeper's signal. OSCEs have been demonstrated to be reliable, valid and feasible, and both examiners and (unusually, perhaps) candidates themselves regard them favourably. However, they do have potential flaws and the organizers need to pay attention to detail because if OSCEs go wrong, they can go disastrously wrong.

The main drawback with OSCEs is the amount of time, space, patients, and examiners they require. They also generate a large quantity of marking sheets and, hence, a large amount of marking. However, the sheets can be designed so that they can be marked by OMR equipment, or the examiners can be asked to total their marks at the end of each candidate's visit to their station, which takes only a few seconds. The marking sheets need to be simple to fill in and the criteria on which marks are awarded must be clearly set out. The item-writers must be careful in identifying the key features of each clinical task they are setting, and the criteria must be based on these features. This will avoid the potential problem of trivializing stations which could result in candidates going through a mental checklist at each one in order to gain marks. Well-constructed OSCEs are an extremely valuable assessment instrument; poorly constructed ones can cause confusion, result in an unreliable examination, or lead to stereotyped behaviour from the candidates. All stations must be field-trialled before they are used in summative OSCEs. (Students are generally pleased to have the opportunity to use new stations formatively and, since there is not an issue of test-security for good OSCE stations, there is no risk of them divulging the answers.)

Another essential feature of a good OSCE is careful training of both examiners and patients. In both instances, this is to ensure that they are well-briefed about the process (and particularly the need to keep to time) and also to ensure consistency in their performance. Of all means of assessing clinical skills, OSCEs have the most to offer when the balance between reliability, validity, and feasibility is considered. The technique is highly applicable to general practice skills, no matter what stage the candidates might have reached, and seems likely to become increasingly common throughout medical education.

31 Assessing communication skills

Lesley Southgate

There is now general agreement amongst medical educators about the importance of learning communication skills as part of undergraduate medical education (Canadian Medical Association 1992). In *Tomorrow's doctors* the Education Committee of the General medical council emphasized that good communication with patients was a core skill for clinicians and this has been discussed previously, especially in Chapters 4 and 14. People have reported the rapid increase of complaints against doctors directed at the quality of the doctor—patient relationship rather than poor clinical skills. However, although there is some evidence (Simpson *et al.* 1991) about the negative effect of poor communication on the outcomes of patient care, some clinicians and life scientists remain unconvinced that a significant amount of time in the curriculum should be devoted to improving the communication skills of medical students. Others pay lip service to such initiatives but undermine them by allowing the students to realize that in their view it is not the really important business of medical education.

Of course, students are interested in the evidence about improved compliance and patient satisfaction that results from good communication. Many acknowledge the benefit of increased confidence in taking the medical history and examining the patient that results from improved communication skills, but they will only practise and think deeply about the area if they know that it will be part of summative assessment, devised and supported by the clinical teachers who act as powerful role models. Hence, the involvement of leading clinicians in the medical school in arguing for assessment of communication skills is vital in persuading reluctant colleagues of the need for change. Once the climate is right the process of developing and implementing the assessment programme can begin; and it begins with a clear statement of the purpose and content before the methods are chosen.

THE PURPOSE AND CONTENT OF COMMUNICATION SKILLS ASSESSMENT

Having established that learning communication skills is a core activity in the undergraduate curriculum both formative and summative assessment must be available to support the learners. The purpose of both types of assessment must be explicit so that students and faculty know exactly how to approach them.

Formative assessment

Formative assessment should be established and available throughout the course to provide feedback and enable the student to assess progress and plan his or her learning. For communication skills this means that students should have opportunities to carry out consultations under direct surveillance (or to have a consultation recorded) and then to work through the consultation with a tutor to consider areas that might be approached differently. This system of assessment should have no implications for the progress of the student although there is a case to be argued for requiring at least a minimum level of participation in the process.

Summative assessment

Summative assessment will happen during or perhaps at the end of the course and has implications for the progress of the student to the next stage or to graduation. A large body of research has shown that assessment drives learning (Newble and Jaeger 1983). That is to say, students study the hidden curriculum (the one that is assessed), and so the inclusion of the assessment of communication skills in summative assessments leads to congruence of the official and hidden curriculum, and ultimately benefits students. Of course, the methods chosen must support the goals and philosophy of the curriculum and reflect the teaching and learning opportunities within it, in other words the assessment methods must demonstrate *consequential validity* (see above, Chapter 28).

CONTENT OF THE CURRICULUM FOR COMMUNICATION SKILLS

Having decided that there will be both formative and summative assessment of communication skills, the next consideration is to determine the circumstances in which a student should be able to communicate well, and the skills that they must demonstrate in those circumstances. This, of course, is part of the much larger work of defining the curriculum, which should be directed at the tasks which a pre-registration doctor should be able to perform, as well as developing lifelong learning skills. It will provide learning opportunities for acquiring skills to carry out these activities and the assessments for whatever purpose will be designed to support this learning. In a modern integrated course there are a number of broad communication skills to be considered such as the ability to communicate in learning groups, the ability to comprehend scientific articles, presentational skills, and the ability to write effectively in lay language. Methods have to be developed to assess each of these. Poster or oral presentations can be marked against set criteria. One approach to assessing more general writing skills has been to present students with a short scientific paper and to ask them to write a précis, taking account of the main scientific points, and then to write an article for a lay magazine or newspaper that uses the essential points of the article. This can be marked against criteria such as ability to determine the key points and to avoid jargon and long words.

The most important area of communication is in the professional area. Undergraduates need to develop communication skills in three areas. They are:

- during the consultation;
- with colleagues while working as a team member;
- through written communication in medical records and letters.

The remainder of this section will chiefly consider the assessment of communication skills within the consultation. However, team-work and written communication are mentioned to encourage their inclusion in future curricula. Assessment of communication skills for team-work has not so far reached prominence in the undergraduate curricula in the United Kingdom, despite the emphasis on team-work in the GMC's *Tomorrow's doctors*. Peer review, structured feedback from other team members, and self-assessment are promising methods for this area which will need considerable research and development as interprofessional education becomes more widespread.

The assessment of written communication can be included as part of in-training assessment, with the records written during clerking reviewed by peers or teachers. It is also possible to include such items as the requirement to write a referral or discharge letter based on a clinical vignette within a written short-answer paper. Pre-registration doctors are expected to make excellent records and to write to colleagues. Poor performance in this area can compromise the standard of care and it is reasonable to expect the undergraduate education should provide opportunities to master and assess the skill.

Communication with patients

What should be the content of the assessment of communication skills with patients? The clinical content areas to be included will derive from the published curriculum, which itself is founded on some notion of the health and illness needs of the population and the variety of the individuals that comprise it. The skills will be those needed to perform the communication tasks of the medical consultation bearing these needs in mind. Most authors agree that these include:

- introductions and attention to ensuring comfort and privacy;
- establishing the reasons for the consultation;
- enabling the patient to tell his or her story;
- introducing the physical examination into the consultation and obtaining consent for it,
- summarizing the patient's story to check accuracy and interpretation;
- explaining the working diagnosis and the proposed management and follow-up;
- seeking the patient's views and agreement on the proposed outcome;
- ending the interview.

Each of these tasks subsumes complex skills, for example, a gynaecological consultation with a non-English speaking Asian woman accompanied by a health advocate requires the additional skills of conducting a consultation with three people present, as well as raising difficulties in almost every one of the above categories. Another example might be a mother with a feverish child, where some of the skills in managing a consultation with three people present may be the same, but the challenge in the different tasks of the consultation will be quite different. In deciding the content areas for assessment of communication all of these dimensions (the needs of the population, the diversity of individuals, the communication tasks of the consultation, the role of the pre-registration doctor) should be used to construct a matrix (blueprint) with realistic boundaries from which the content can be sampled. Every student will have access to this document which should be part of the overall blueprint for assessment.

It is a counter-intuitive but unarguable research finding that demonstrating clinical competence and performance in one content area does not predict it in another (van der Vleuten *et al*. 1991). There has been relatively little research on the generalizability of communication skills as an entity separate from the clinical content of cases but the evidence so far indicates that performance in one content area is not necessarily correlated with performance in another (Hodges *et al*. 1994). In other words, the ability to communicate the result of a positive HIV test does not predict the ability to tell a patient she has breast cancer. This means that while improvements in methods to assess communication skills are awaited, any programme of assessment must sample a wide area of clinical content in order to achieve reproducible results.

METHODS FOR ASSESSING COMMUNICATION SKILLS

The choice of methods follows clarification of the purpose and definition of the content and should support the development of adult learning skills. The same methods may be used for different purposes provided that the students are informed beforehand.

Assessing knowledge of communication skills

There is a case to be made for assessing the understanding of the basic concepts of communication skills by inclusion of items in written knowledge tests. This would be at an elementary level and could be provided in the format of extended matching items for use soon after the students start seeing patients (e.g. short excerpts of transcripts of actual interviews could be matched to lists of skills).

Direct observation of the encounter

The best way to assess communication skills is by observing them during the consultaion, whether it be in general practice or a hospital setting. There are a variety of ways of achieving this aim which can be used in any combination:

- An observer may be present or view through a one-way mirror, or the interview may be recorded on audio or videotape.
- The interview may be with a real or standardized patient.

- The interview may be in a real or simulated setting.
- The assessment may be done by the student (self), peers, examiners, or real or standardized patients.

In an assessment, formative or summative, conducted using any combination of these strategies, it is imperative that all of the participants, especially real patients and students, give informed consent to what is proposed. The written consent of patients for observed or recorded consultations should be obtained and kept with their medical records and the audio or videotape according to GMC guidelines (1994; see Chapter 14, Fig. 14.1).

The use of standardized patients

Standardized patients have been discussed in Chapter 14. They are individuals trained to function as patients and sometimes as teachers and assessors (Stillman *et al.* 1986, 1991). They can be asymptomatic, or present symptoms, and some have stable physical signs on examination such as heart murmurs, hernias, or joint abnormalities. Sometimes they can simulate various physical findings such as deep abdominal tenderness or diminished breath sounds and they can simulate different personalities and moods. Standardized patients are trained to reproducibly and realistically portray patients, and Rethans and colleagues (1991) showed that experienced doctors behave in a similar way with standardized patients as with real patients, and cannot detect the difference when standardized patients arrive unannounced in a general practice. Standardized patients can themselves assess every aspect of the consultation by completing checklists or rating scales and can be a valuable resource for formative assessment and for educational-needs assessment (van der Vleuten and Swanson 1990). There is an increasing tendency world-wide to use standardized patients in summative examinations both at the undergraduate and postgraduate level (Vu *et al.* 1992; Grand Maison *et al.* 1992; Bingham *et al.* 1994) although their use as sole raters in these circumstances is still not allowed by the university regulations governing some UK medical schools.

The information completed by the standardized patient after the consultation may be specific to the case content or generic as in communication skills. There are a large number of instruments available or under development (Petrusa *et al.* 1995; Schnabl *et al.* 1991): those which relate to communication skills all enable the standardized patient to record the sensitivity and rapport that was established, the degree to which the patient was involved in decisions, and the adequacy of explanations. As the use of standardized patients becomes more widespread in UK undergraduate examinations, evidence about the content and reliability of scales or checklists will emerge.

The use of standardized patients for teaching in the United Kingdom has led to the establishment of groups of trained individuals associated with several medical schools. The development of patient roles for assessment will be a priority as the use of the OSCE is taken up for summative assessments of both clinical and consulting skills. The roles are usually based on clinical cases from the experience of the clinicians charged with ensuring the content validity and level of difficulty of the assessment. Training for the standardized patient comprises immersion in the patient-focused material about the case which may be written, or in the innovative approach developed by Rashid *et al.* (1994) in Leicester, includes a videotape of a consultation by the actual patient on whom the case is based. In some standardized patient groups the training is done by non-clinical group members, in others medical school faculty conduct it. In any case, it is important to test the cases with faculty and students before including them in the bank of roles for use in formative and summative assessment.

Self-assessment

Self-assessment of communication skills is a useful formative experience. Usually, it involves the student watching a videotaped interview alone and using a checklist or scale to rate the performance. Students are usually much more critical of themselves than other raters and it is often of benefit to have other ratings done independently to demonstrate this to them (see below, *assessment by peers*). The ability to rate oneself is an important part of adult learning (Hays 1990) and this is one of the reasons for including it in the undergraduate curriculum. One school in the United Kingdom includes self-assessment of communication skills, based on a written critique of a transcribed audiotaped interview, in a mandatory in-training assessment at the end of the clinical introductory course (Jolly *et al.* 1994). There is some evidence that students in problem-based medical schools are more accurate in self-assessment although the reasons for the association are not yet clear (MacFadyen and Turnbull 1995)

Assessment by peers

Assessment by peers either in groups or individually is another valuable approach. Students are usually very careful with each other, although they must be given the skills to provide constructive feedback in giving the results of assessments to their colleagues. Innovation in assessment will certainly include a formative peer assessment programme for clinical and consulting skills, real innovation will extend this approach to summative assessment.

External assessment

Assessment by examiner/assessors is used in the United Kingdom more than is necessary, in that much of it could probably be done by standardized patients. Where teachers and clinicians do act as examiners, and this is usually in summative assessments, they must receive information and training in order to optimize reliability of the scores. There are several instruments developed for postgraduate general practice which may have relevance to the undergraduate curriculum, but their use in undergraduate summative examinations has not yet been reported in the literature (Campbell *et al.* 1995; Cox and Mulholland 1993; Fraser *et al.* 1994). Where teachers are involved in formative assessment of communication skills they should be trained in the use of any scales or checklists, be able to give constructive feedback, and have tried the approach on themselves before they use it with the students.

Standard setting

Standard setting for these assessments is of great importance if they are to be used for summative purposes with great care taken to define the criteria against which the student is to be judged. These will be different for different levels of experience and will also determine the way in which students approach formative assessment. Components of communication, such as enabling or summarizing can be tested in shorter OSCE stations, but greater validity is achieved by assessing a complete interview in a reasonable amount of time (say 10 minutes) with a minimum of 18 standardized patient interviews or 180 minutes of testing time needed for content validity and adequate reliability for summative assessments. The rules for pass/fail decisions and the criteria for awarding scores are decided by detailed consideration of each case by the relevant clinical and communication experts.

32 Guidelines for assessing clinical competence

Lesley Southgate

The assessment of competence, what the student 'knows how' to do, is the task of all those who develop and engage in the undergraduate curriculum. It is important for the support of students as they graduate and enter the world of work, it is important for the public who are protected via the requirements of the GMC and it is important for the teachers and learners in the medical school who will suffer frustration and disappointment if the assessed hidden curriculum and the published taught curriculum are not congruent.

There are several principles that should be followed by those who devise the assessments for undergraduate education which should be coordinated throughout the medical school rather than be based in departments or disciplines. This is of particular importance as vertical and horizontal integration and problem based approaches are adopted. If appropriate assessments are not developed from the beginning, innovation will be stifled. It should be clear that an overall approach to assessment has been proposed. In particular assessment should not start with choosing the methods first! The following guidelines provide a basis for those who are concerned with test development.

GUIDELINES (Newble 1993)

* *Decide and publish the purpose of the assessments*:
  – summative, formative, progress test.

* *Define the content*:
  – based on the clinical problems that a pre-registration doctor must be able to resolve and the things the doctor should know or be able to do on graduation.

* *Prepare a blueprint for sampling the content systematically*.
* *Select the test methods*:
  – tests should represent reality (fidelity), they should be appropriate to the task that is posed, practical constraints must be recognized;
  – pay attention to reliability and validity, an unreliable assessment is inherently invalid. Combine different methods into a test battery to maximize effectiveness and efficiency.

- *Scoring*:
  - develop marking schedules ahead of the examination and use them,
  - use pre-tested scales or checklists,
  - take care in combining scores and ensure that each component contributes its intended weight to the overall result,
  - avoid bias based on such factors as gender and ethnicity.

- *Standard setting*:
  - standards are best criterion-referenced for undergraduate summative assessments. Involve content experts, students and educationalists in this process.

- *Reporting scores*:
  - this should allow the maximum feedback for students, general feedback for faculty on which to base course improvements, information to the medical school to allow the decision to be made on whether the student can graduate, and information to the GMC for the purposes of the register.

- *Staff development*:
  - institute a programme of faculty development to ensure that there is an understanding of the tasks of the assessment committee and the staff and students in relation to assessments.

- *Resources*:
  - secure a budget for all of the activities related to assessments to be held by the group responsible for assessments. Examinations and formative assessments are expensive and cannot be subsumed into departmental budgets.

33 Evaluating the curriculum

Gareth Holsgrove

Evaluating teaching is an important part of the curriculum evaluation process, but not the only part. The content, timing, duration, assessment, feedback to students (and tutors), and a number of other aspects of the curriculum must also be evaluated. It is important to look beyond an evaluation of teaching when the curriculum features self-directed learning. In this situation, formal teaching may be almost totally absent, but it is intended that a considerable amount of learning will occur. The course leader will also be interested in evaluation of new elements of the course particularly now that there is a much greater emphasis on quality assurance. There are two perspectives on teaching that those responsible for organizing or working on a course will need to know about. The first is what the students feel about it; the second, how the staff see their own teaching.

STUDENT OPINION

Student opinion can be sampled, summarized in report form, and distributed quite widely. However, it is strongly recommended that critical comments do not identify any specific individual by name in published versions (although they can appear in a 'confidential' report to the person in charge of the course). On the other hand, tutors whose work is praised will normally be very pleased to see their efforts recognized by the students and they should certainly be named.

Although a quick survey of student opinion can be conducted by a simple show of hands, more useful results can be obtained by using questionnaires. In either case, however, it is important that the questions are prepared with some care. They should also be fairly specific, although space can be left on questionnaires for additional comments.

Questionnaires can be given to all of the students, or just to a random sample. They are easier to deal with, however, if they are relatively short and quick to fill in. Multiple pages tend to get in a mess, and students' enthusiasm might wane after the first few items. Probably the quickest way to obtain useful information is to base the items on a Likert-type scale. This should have at least 5 points but not exceed 7. A 6-point scale is useful if the evaluator wants to avoid a 'neutral' mid-point. When evaluating qualitative issues (e.g. 'How clear were the explanations?') then the highest number on the scale should represent the best rating (i.e. 'very clear') and the lowest (1) the worst ('very confusing'). It is best to avoid using zero as the lowest point because it can then be difficult to discriminate zero responses from those which have been omitted.

Questions about quantitative topics can also be answered on a similar scale. In these cases, it is suggested that only a 5-or 7-point scale is used because a mid-point is needed. A question asking, for example, about the number of lectures in the course, would receive a response of a high number if the student felt that there were 'far too many', a mid-point response if they felt the number of lectures 'about right', and a low number if there were felt to be 'too few' lectures.

One interesting innovation in the curriculum evaluation of a new course at St Bartholomew's and the Royal London School of Medicine and Dentistry was the use of the University of London TFQ answer sheets for student responses. This enabled the forms to be scanned by the central computer equipment and the results from virtually a whole intake of students (around 300) to be available within a few hours.

TUTORS' SELF-EVALUATION

Curriculum evaluation is still not routine, although it is becoming much more common. Asking tutors to assess their own performance is rare and, because it is also potentially very threatening, must be approached with care. However, it can be a very useful process. At first, it is probably essential to keep tutors' personal evaluations totally private. Although they may feel free to discuss them if they wish, there must be no obligation to do this. However, if they do choose to discuss them, it may be particularly helpful if this is done along with the students' evaluation of their teaching. Used in this way, it may serve as a confidence booster for good tutors who are over-critical of their own work. It may also help to identify reasons why a tutor who thinks they are doing a good job obtains poor evaluations from the students.

Tutors' self-evaluation may begin by addressing just a few key points:

- Had I planned the session adequately?
- If not, what will I improve next time?
- Did I cover all the objectives I had planned to?
- Did I summarize adequately?
- Do I think the students achieved anything as a result of the session?
- Did the students seem to find it interesting?
- What were the main good points about this teaching session? (make a note and be sure to use them again).
- What are the main points I should like to improve? (make a note and be sure to improve them).

If the session was a lecture or similar presentation then the following may be additional points to address:

- Did I present my material in a clear, logical order?

- Could everybody hear me?
- Did I have audio/visual aids? (if not, do I need them?)
- Were my audio/visual aids audible/visible? (and were they appropriate?)
- Did I allow sufficient time for questions?

Tutors may like to consider devising a similar series of additional questions for one-to-one sessions and for small group sessions, especially problem-based sessions where a good facilitator may sometimes be the quietest person in the room!

As tutors become more familiar with this process, they are likely to find it a helpful one and, one hopes, the quality of their work will improve. If it does, tutors' confidence will increase and they might introduce new elements into their self-evaluation strategy.

Part Six
Conclusion

Time present and time past
Are both perhaps present in time future,
And time future contained in time past.
(T.S.Eliot 1989, The *four quartets*, Burnt Norton I)

It is unlikely that many people a few years ago could have foreseen the way that general practice in the United Kingdom would develop in the last decade of the 20th century. The Alma—Ata Declaration was a resounding clarion call to think in terms of primary health care. Yet, in many ways, it seemed to be talking to the poor and developing countries rather than those that had developed a highly sophisticated technical approach to medical care. The concept of a primary care-led NHS was far from the minds of those who rejoiced in the therapeutic and technological revolutions in medicine. Continually there were exciting new advances from powerful diagnostic imaging to the ability to replace worn-out parts. The need seemed to be for people who could spearhead these advances with powerful scientific brains. But, simultaneously, the echoes of many teachers, from Hippocrates to William Osler, sounded a warning that medical care which started to treat people out of context in remote 'disease palaces' would fail to provide for the real needs of its patients. The general public were becoming more aware of what might be done and how it might be done. Patients knew that their suffering was much more complex than the physical or mental ailments they suffered. They might demand the antibiotics, but at the same time they resented the lack of empathy that accompanied the prescription.

Many factors have begun to change the situation in Western countries. Economic realities have forced governments to think how health care can be provided in the most cost-effective way. In the UK, at least, it appears that good primary care is important in this. Communities are waking up and demanding more knowledge and more say in the running of their services. Educational bodies have been forced to radically rethink the nature of their input and have been open to new attitudes and new approaches. The scientific community is more open to new paradigms and 'truth' is no longer limited to a reductionist bioscience that tries to explain everything in molecular terms.

Community-based medical education is one way to bring the doctors of the future face to face with many of these issues. There is, however, a danger summed up in the saying: 'A revolution is so-called because it goes full circle'. If the changes currently taking place in medical education are to lead to further advances, it is necessary to think about them critically and to start to consider what the next stages should be. In this final section two short chapters consider these issues and suggest an agenda for some areas that merit consideration in the 21st century.

34 Demonstrating the benefits

For a long time it was considered unnecessary to look at the benefits of teaching activity. If students passed their examinations, that was enough. No one asked whether this was because of good and appropriate teaching, or whether it was because there were good textbooks available! More recently there has been an increased emphasis on the quality of the teaching and this was considered in Chapter 33. There is a danger that such feedback can be superficial. Too many students' questionnaires ask little more than whether the session was interesting and useful (for what?). Avoiding evaluation or superficial approaches to it are no longer acceptable. Furthermore, the outcome must be considered as well as the process. A major redeployment of educational resources into the community should be based on two bits of evidence that demonstrate the benefits:

- The end-product must be better-suited to the needs of the health care system.
- The educational process must have been important in achieving that end-product.

In the past, the teaching hospitals in the United Kingdom have received considerable financial resources for their educational work. They will not let these go lightly.

Demonstrating the benefits will be a complex task. Since it takes at least nine years from entry to medical school to being a vocationally trained general practitioner (and longer for other specialties), it is a long process to prove that the end-product of new systems is better. It is necessary to set the agenda now.

THE COMPETENCE OF THE DOCTOR

It will have been noted that in Part V there was a focus on knowledge and clinical skills (including communication). These are the keys to assessing competence in terms of what a doctor should know or be able to do on graduation. However, as has been seen, the General Medical Council has also put considerable emphasis on attitudes (the affective domain). Many of these areas (e.g. person-centredness or ability to cope with uncertainty) are central to the input from the community. If the benefits of community input are to be shown, it will be necessary to address the question of attitudinal assessment. There are major problems here, ranging from what is an acceptable attitude to how feasible it is to test it. There is anyway an underlying question as to the extent to which attitudes can be changed by education! In determining the benefits of community education the following issues will need to be addressed:

- Can attitudinal objectives be clearly defined?
- Can measurable outcomes be stated?
- Might the outcomes conflict with equal opportunities (and similar) legislation?
- Who are the most appropriate assessors: other doctors, other health professionals or patients/lay people?
- Can change in attitudes be demonstrated?

THE EFFECTIVENESS OF THE DOCTOR

Although the newly trained doctors may fit the guidelines produced by the GMC, the question will remain whether they are acceptable to the public and able to deliver what the public needs. In the last decade of the 20th century there has been a crisis of confidence in the health professionals with many people becoming disillusioned and demotivated. There have been marked recruitment problems, not least in primary care. Although medicine is still a high-status profession with many people wanting to enter it at the age of 18, there is a considerable loss of enthusiasm at a later stage. Often this is because the doctors feel that they are not effective or that patients do not respond to them. The effective doctor is not only one who is competent and able to demonstrate all the right attitudes of patient-centredness; the effective doctor is one who is recognized by the community as providing for their needs. There can be a conflict here as was shown in Chapter 15. Resolving this conflict may require that patients are involved in many more aspects of medical education. The community, where patients can be found who are articulate and active, may be the best source of such people. The following issues need to be addressed if we are to have effective doctors:

- Can patients be involved in the selection of students for medical school?
- Can patients be involved in the planning of curricula?
- Can patients be involved in the education of students?
- Can patients be involved in the assessment of students?

THE EFFECTIVENESS OF THE EDUCATION

The third item on the agenda is to demonstrate that education in the community can be delivered enjoyable, economically, and effectively. Students have usually enjoyed brief attachments to general practices, particularly appreciating the one-to-one teaching. Self-selected students have shown how they have enjoyed the long attachment in the Cambridge Community-based Clinical Course (Wharton 1995). However, both students and hospital doctors will need to be convinced that the longer spells in the community for everyone are worthwhile. There will be many difficulties for students: travelling will increase, they may be isolated more from their peers, and they will find they have to search out more learning opportunities for themselves. It will be easy for poor teaching to produce very negative reactions. It will be very important to determine which aspects of community-based medical education are important in achieving objectives. As skills laboratories, computer-assisted learning (CAL) and other institution-based approaches develop, it may be that some of the advantages of community placements will be less obvious. It will be very important to make sure that the time spent in the community is effectively used to achieve objectives that cannot be more economically achieved elsewhere.

The following issues must be considered:

- How will the new teaching approaches be monitored?
- How well are objectives related to resources?
- Is it possible to compare the results of assessments of students taught by the new methods and those taught traditionally?

CONCLUSION

This chapter has taken a brief look at some issues involved in demonstrating that there are benefits in the move to community-based education. It will also be necessary to show that these benefits can actually be delivered. The new approaches to financing teaching include plans for monitoring the quality. This will be an essential task, although in itself it will require considerable resource. The similar situation in vocational training in general practice has shown the value of time spent on selecting, accrediting, and re-accrediting training practices. Undergraduate education will need to follow the same road. Tutors should not find this a threat, but rather a challenge to produce an end-product medical graduate who will be competent, effective, and well motivated to work with them in the health service of the 21st century.

35 Changing education in the 21st century

The current wave of curricular change is not limited to the United Kingdom. Similar developments are occurring all over the world. The status, purpose, and nature of doctors is changing, especially as other health care professions develop. Nursing and many other professions now have university-based courses, often using very similar educational approaches. As this stage of the educational revolution gathers momentum, it will be necessary to look beyond to some of the next wave of challenges that will affect the process.

INTEGRATING THE DOCTORS

Integrated courses and moving education into the community are still at an early stage. Multidisciplinary teaching is in its infancy: often, people from different disciplines come to a session with the single aim of providing an input from their own perspective. It is frequently difficult to get a group of tutors together in advance to plan a session, to decide who is going to be the lead tutor, and who are going to act as resources and, at the end, how a joint assessment can be made. Too often this process means that students get a fragmented message. This may be the way the 'real world' is, but is not a good role model for the future. Community tutors are going to need to work with their hospital colleagues to develop effective joint-teaching and to demonstrate the new 'seamless' health service. One aspect of this is ensuring that a single message is given in areas where many different disciplines necessarily have input. A good example is communication skills. Hospital doctors are keenly aware of the importance of these, but often find it hard to work with community colleagues to teach them in an integrated way.

As community-based teaching moves from being an isolated attachment to being an integral part of the curriculum, it should be seen as just one resource among many. The tutors will need to meet together to plan, train, and assess.

INTEGRATING UNDERGRADUATE AND POSTGRADUATE EDUCATION

The radical changes that are taking place in undergraduate education will soon have a major effect on education in the postgraduate sphere. Adult learners who have spent much of their time being self-motivated enquirers will want the facilities to continue that approach. The days of lunchtime lectures in sleepy postgraduate centres are probably numbered. Information will be available through the 'information highway'. What will be required will be skills in assessing and using it. It is likely that distance learning, teleconferencing, and small interest groups on the Internet will play an increasing role in developing and maintaining knowledge and skills. These will be available for doctors in their workplace and homes.

Specialist training is changing radically with the introduction of the Specialist Registrar Grade. The specialist colleges are beginning to review their assessment procedures and introducing elements such as assessment of communication skills. The need for this will be greater as patients themselves have greater access to the knowledge base, and clinicians have to consider how to explain their reasoning processes and negotiate plans. This will require greater emphasis on the individual and contextual elements of diagnosis by all doctors. The community must surely continue to have a major role to play in this. The move towards pre-registration house-officer posts in the community is already gaining momentum. All these changes could make considerable demands on community tutors and consideration will need to be given again to what elements of education demand access to community resources.

INTEGRATING THE PRACTICE TEAM

Throughout this book, the concept of multiprofessional training has been put forward. It is clear this is currently in its infancy but it is likely to come to the forefront over the next generation. In some universities, dentists and doctors already share the first years of training. Other health professions may well become involved in this. At first sight the development of vertically integrated medical courses might seem to conflict with the concept of a basic 'health sciences' course to be followed by further professional training in medicine, nursing, physiotherapy, etc. However, there will be many professional and economic factors that will promote the idea. Already, the need to share the perspectives of different health professions in understanding the process of clinical reasoning has been seen (Higgs and Jones 1996). As professional boundaries blur and the status of many non-medical health professions increases, so it will become evident that these different professions need increasing amount of joint contact. Many learning needs will be the same and it will become evident that educational resources should be shared.

Meanwhile, general practices will be providing a considerable amount of multipro-fessional input. Other professionals in the practice (such as practice managers and practice nurses) will play an increasing role as educational resources for students. It is likely that the administrative staff within a practice will organize much of the teaching. This means they need to understand why different activities are going on. These staff will require some input to develop these roles. Medical tutors will need to be aware of this. A major challenge for the future will be to develop a practice in its entirety as a training resource to provide a very different style of teaching.

INTEGRATING WITH PATIENTS

The part played by patients in the whole educational role has been increasingly emphasized in this book. There is no doubt that patients can often be the most effective tutors. In the past, much of this contact has been arranged haphazardly. In future, practices should think how patients can be more effectively integrated into the teaching team. Some hospitals have already developed lists of patients in the community who can be called on for particular teaching sessions. A similar approach has been used in initiatives like the King's Medical Firm in the Community (Chapter 20). Teaching practices should consider how to organize this. It may well be that a practice patients' group would wish to initiate this on its own.

Health care facilities are likely to develop in the 21st century in many new ways. There will be different approaches to health promotion, out-of-hours centres, walk-in advice in pharmacies, health shops, mental health centres, drug drop-ins, and so on. People involved in these, often lay people, will be very interested in having contact with medical students. It may well be that Community Health Councils, local Councils of Voluntary Service and other similar organizations will want to come together to provide a stronger lay input into medical education as has been found in London (see Chapters 17 and 18). There are copious resources within communities who are concerned with supporting and caring for people: students can benefit from spending time with them but the organization is a major challenge

INTEGRATING INTERNATIONALLY

The medical elective has long been an opportunity for people to work in a different health care system. Many students are radically changed by the experience. With the developments of the European Union there is an increasing flow of students and graduates across national boundaries. Some universities are already initiating a combined medical degree with European studies: the students will spend a large part of the course at a European university. Seeing the ways that different national cultures have approached the provision of health care helps students to broaden their understanding of health beliefs and can also instil a critically analytical approach to many medical interventions. Considerable benefits might be obtained by encouraging an increasing amount of international educational travel. Students should be able to spend time in other national communities, and not just in the slightly rarefied atmosphere of the hospitals.

CONCLUSION

Experience and reflection have been key principles in the consideration of how to teach medicine in the community. The broader the experience, the better the opportunities for effective reflection. As students face the challenges of the 21st century in the increasingly multicultural societies of the global village, they will need a wide understanding of what illness means. They also need to experience how people work together to confront suffering and misery: not only doctors of many disciplines, but also an ever-increasing group of other professionals; not only health professionals, but also the lay public. A good community-based education will provide this and will also open up the powers of reflection.

References

Ashton, J. and Seymour H. (1988). *The new public health*. Open University Press, Milton Keynes.

Balarajan, R. and Soni Raleigh, V. (1992). The ethnic populations of England and Wales: the 1991 Census. *Health Trends*, **24**, 113–16.

Barrows, H.S. and Tamblyn, R.M. (1980). *Problem-based learning: An approach to medical education*. Springer, New York.

Belbin, R.M. (1981). *Management Teams: Why they succeed or fail*. Heinemann, London.

Bingham, E., Burrows, P., *et al.* (1994). Simulated surgery: a framework for the assessment of clinical competence. *Education for General Practice*, **5**, 143–50.

Bligh, J. (1995). Problem based, small group learning: an idea whose time has come. *British Medical Journal*, **311**, 342–3.

Bloom, B.S. (ed.) (1965). *Taxonomy of educational objectives—The classification of educational goals*. Handbook I, *The cognitive domain*. Longman, New York.

Boud, D. (ed.) (1985). *Reflection: Turning experience into learning*. Kogan Page, London.

Bowmer, I., Davis, W., des Marchais, J., Gabb, R., Norcini, J., and Whelan G. (1994). Standard setting in certification tests. In *The certification and recertification of doctors: Issues in the assessment of clinical competence*, (ed. D.Newble, B.Jolly, and R.Wakeford) Cambridge University Press.

BMA (British Medical Association) (1995). *Report of the working party on medical education*. BMA, London.

Byrne, P.S. (1973). University departments of general practice and the undergraduate teaching of general practice in the United Kingdom in 1972. *Journal of the Royal College of General Practitioners*, **23**, (Suppl. 1).

Byrne, P.S. and Long, B.E.L. (1975). *Learning to care: Person to person*. Churchill Livingstone, Edinburgh.

Campbell, L., Howie, J., and Murray, S. (1995). Use of videotaped consultations in summative assessment of trainees in general practice. *British Journal of General Practice*. **45**, 137–41.

Campion, P.D., Stanley, I.M., and Haddleton, M. (1992). Audit in general practice: students and practitioners learning together. *Quality in Health Care*, **1**, 114–18

Canadian Medical Association (1992). Consensus statement from the Workshop on Teaching and Assessment of Communication Skills in Canadian Medical Schools. *Canadian Medical Association Journal*, **147**, 8.

Case, S.M. and Swanson, D.B. (1992). *Item writing guide*. National Board of Medical Examiners, Philadelphia, PA.

Chronbach, L.J., Gleser, G.C., Harinder Nanda, A.N, and Rajaratnam, N. (1972). *The dependability of behavioural measurements: theory of generalisability for scores and profiles.* Wiley, New York.

Chugh, U., Dillman, E., Kurtz, S.M., Lockyer, J., and Parboosingh, J. (1993). Multicultural issues in medical curriculum: implications for Canadian physicians. *Medical Teacher*, **15**, 83–91.

Cohen, H. (1954). The balanced curriculum. In *Proceedings of the First World Conference on Medical Education.* Geoffrey Cumberlege, Oxford University Press, London

Coles, C.R. (1990). Elaborated learning in undergraduate medical education. *Medical Education*, **24**, 14–22.

Coles, C.R. (1994). A review of learner-centred education and its applications in primary care. *Education for General Practice*, **5**, 19–25.

Cox, J. and Mulholland, H. (1993). An instrument for assessment of videotapes of general practitioners performance. *British Medical Journal*, **306**, 1043–6.

David, T.J. and Patel, L. (1995). Adult learning theory, problem based learning, and paediatrics. *Archives of Disease in Childhood*, **73**, 357–63.

de Groot, L. (1987). Pliable but not receptive: concerning the marginal influence of a medical psychology course on the socialization process of doctors. *Medical Education*, **21**, 419–425.

Denicolo, P., Entwistle N, and Hounsell D. (1992). *Effective learning and teaching in higher education.* Module 1, *What is active learning?* CVCP Universities' Staff Development and Training Unit, Sheffield.

Department of Health (1992). *The health of the nation: A strategy for health in England* HMSO (Cm.1986), London.

Donaldson, R.J. and Donaldson, I.J. (1993). *Essential public health medicine.* Kluwer Academic Press, London.

Dowrick, C., Graham-Jones, S., and Stanley, I. (1992). Mental health in the community. *Medical Education*, **26**, 145–52.

Eisenbruch, M. (1989). Medical education for a multicultural society. *Medical Journal of Australia*, **151**, 574–80.

Eliot, T.S. (1959). *The four quartets.* Faber, London. Engel, C. (1992). Problem-based learning. *British Journal of Hospital Medicine*, **48**, 325–9.

Ellis, J. (1986). *L H M C 1785–1985: The story of England's first medical school.* London Hospital Medical Club, London.

Engel, G.L. (1980). The clinical application of the biopsychosocial model. *American Journal of Psychiatry*, **137**, 535–44.

Engel, G.L. (1992). Problem based learning. *British Journal of Hospital Medicine*, **48**, 325–29.

Ewing, J. (1916). Principles and experiments in medical education, *JAMA*, **66**, 635.

Fairhurst, K., Stanley, I., and Griffiths, C. (1995). Should medical students learn more about management? *British Journal of General Practice*, **45**, 2–3.

Fleming, P.R. (1988). The profitability of 'guessing' in multiple choice question papers. *Medical Education*, **22**, 509–13.

Flexner A. (1912). *Medical Education in europe.* Carnegie Foundation, New York.

Fraser, R., McKinley, R., and Mulholland, H. (1994). Consultation competence in general practice: establishing the face validity of prioritized criteria in the Leicester assessment package. *British Journal of General Practice*, **44**, 109–13.

GMC (General Medical Council) (1987). *Recommendations on training of specialists.* GMC, London.

GMC (General Medical Council.) (1993). *Tomorrow's doctors: Recommendations on undergraduate medical education.* GMC, London.

GMC (General Medical Council) (1995). *News Review.*

Gill, P.S. and Adshead, D. (1996). Teaching cultural aspects of health: a vital part of communication. *Medical Teacher,* **18**, 61–4.

Gillon, R. (1985). *Philosophical medical ethics.* Wiley, Chichester.

Graham, H.J. and Seabrook, M. (1995). Structured packs for independent learning in the community. *Medical Education,* **29**, 61–4.

Goldbeck-Wood, S. (1996). Choosing tomorrow's doctors. *British Medical Journal,* **313**, 313–14.

Grand 'Maison, P., Lescop, J., and Rainsberry, P. (1992). Large-scale use of an objective structured clinical examination for licensing family physicians. *Canadian Medical Association Journal,* **146**, 1735–40.

Griffiths, S. and Partington, P. (1992). *Effective learning and teaching in higher education.* Module 5, *Enabling active learning in small groups.* CVCP Universities' Staff Development and Training Unit, Sheffield.

Hamilton, J.D. (1992). A community and population-oriented medical school: Newcastle, Australia. In *The medical school's mission and the population's health,* (ed. K.L. White and J.E.Connelly). Springer, New York.

Harden, R.M. and Gleeson, F.A. (1979). Assessment of clinical competence using an objective structured clinical examination. *Medical Education,* **13**, 41–54.

Harden, R.M., Stevenson, M., Downie, W.W., and Wilson, G.M. (1975). Assessment of clinical competence using objective structured examination. *British Medical Journal,* **i**, 447–51.

Hays, R. (1990). Self-evaluation of videotaped consultations. *Teaching and Learning in Medicine,* **2**, 232–6.

Heavey, A. (1988). Learning to talk with patients. *British Journal of Hospital Medicine,* **39**, 533–8.

HMSO (Her Majesty's Stationery Office) (1987). *Promoting better health: The government's programme for improving primary health care.* HMSO (Cm. 249), London.

HMSO (Her Majesty's Stationery Office) (1989*a*). *Working for patients.* HMSO (Cm. 555), London.

HMSO (Her Majesty's Stationery Office) (1989*b*). *Caring for people: Community care in the next decade and beyond.* HMSO (Cm. 849), London.

Higgs, J. and Jones, M. (ed.) (1996). *Clinical reasoning in the health professions.* Butterworth-Heinemann, Oxford.

Hodges, B., Turnbull, J., Cohen, R., *et al.* (1994). Assessment of communication skills with complex cases using an OSCE format. In *Proceedings of the Sixth Ottawa Conference on Medical Education,* (ed. A. Rothman and R. Cohen). University of Toronto Bookstore Custom Publishing, Toronto.

Holsgrove, G.J. (1992). Guide to postgraduate exams: multiple choice questions. *British Journal of Hospital Medicine,* **48**, 757–761.

Holsgrove, G.J. (1994). Multiple choice questions in UK medical education. In *Proceedings of the Sixth Ottawa Conference on Medical Education,* (ed. A. Rothman and R. Cohen). University of Toronto Bookstore Custom Publishing, Toronto.

Hopkins, A. and Bahl, V.(ed.) (1993). *Access to health care for people from black and ethnic minorities.* The Royal College of Physicians, London.

Irvine, D. (1972). *Teaching practices. Report from general Practice,* 15. Royal College of General Practitioners, London.

Jolly, B. (1976). Guessing in multiple choice questions. *Medical Education,* **10**, 530.

Jolly, B., Cushing, A., and Dacre, J. (1994). Reliability and validity of a patient-based workbook for assessment of clinical and communication skills. In *Proceedings of the Sixth Ottawa*

Conference on Medical Education, (ed. A. Rothman and R. Cohen). University of Toronto Bookstore Custom Publishing, Toronto.

King, M. (1966). *Medical care in developing countries*. Oxford University Press Nairobi.

Ley, P. (1988). *Communicating with patients*. Chapman & Hall, London.

Light, D. (1979), Uncertainty and control in professional training. *Journal of Health and Social Behaviour*, **20**, 310–22.

Livingston, S.A. and Zicky, M.J. (1982). *Passing scores: a manual for setting standards of performance on educational and occupational tests*. Educational Testing Service, Princeton.

Lyons, A.S. and Petrucelli R.J. (1987). *Medicine: An illustrated history*. Abrams, New York.

MacFadyen, J. and Turnbull, J. (1994). Effect of curriculum on student self-assessment of communication skills. In *Proceedings of the Sixth Ottawa Conference on Medical Education*, (ed. A. Rothman and R. Cohen). University of Toronto Bookstore Custom Publishing, Toronto.

Marinker, M. (ed) (1990). *Medical audit in general practice*. British Medical Association, London.

Marteau, T.M., Humphrey, C., Matoon, G., Kidd, J., Lloyd, M., and Horder, J. (1991). Factors influencing the communication skills of first-year clinical medical students. *Medical Education*, **25**, 127–34.

Mayo, W.J. (1928). National Education Association: Proceedings and addresses, **66**, 163.

McCormick, J. (1992). The contribution of general practice. In *The making of a doctor*. (ed. R.S. Downie and B. Charlton). Oxford University Press.

McCrorie, P., Lefford, F., and Perrin, F. (1993) *Medical undergraduate community-based teaching: A survey for ASME on current and proposed teaching in the community and in general practice in U.K. Universities*. ASME, Dundee.

Metz, J.C.M., Stoelinga, G.B.A., Pels Rijcken-Van Erp Taalman Kip, E.H., and van den Brand-Valkenburg, B.W.M. (1994). *Blueprint 1994: Training of doctors in the Netherlands*. University of Nijmegen, The Netherlands.

Mitchell, K., Haynes, R., and Koenig J (1994). Assessing the validity of the updated medical-college admission test. *Academic Medicine*, **69**, 393–401.

Monekosso, G.L. (1993). The teaching of medicine at the University Centre for Health Sciences, Yaounde, Cameroon: Its concordance with the Edinburgh Declaration on Medical Education. *Medical Education*, **27**, 304–320.

Newble, D. and Entwhistle, N. (1986). Learning styles and approaches: implications for medical education. *Medical Education*, **20**, 162–75.

Newble, D. (ed.) (1983). Guidelines for the development of effective and efficient procedures for the assessment of clinical competence. In *The certification and recertification of doctors: Issues in the assessment of clinical competence*, (ed. D.Newble, B.Jolly, and R.Wakeford). Cambridge University Press.

Newble, D. and Jaeger, K. (1983). The effect of assessments and examinations on the learning of medical students. *Medical Education*, **17**, 165–71.

Norman, G.R. (1988). Problem-solving skills, solving problems and problem-based learning. *Medical Education*, **22**, 279–86.

Osler, W. (1951) The student life. In *A way of life and selected writings of Sir William Osler*. Dover, New York.

Oswald, N. (1989). Why not base clinical education in general practice? *Lancet*, **ii**, 148–9.

Oswald, N. and Jones, S. (1994). Medical students in general practice. *British Journal of General Practice*, **44**, 184–5.

Oswald, N., Jones, S., Date, J., and Hinds, D. (1995). Long term community-based attachments: the Cambridge Course. *Medical Education*, **29**, 72–6.

Pendleton, D.A., Schofield, T.P.C., Tate, P., and Havelock, P.B. (1984). *The consultation*: An *approach to learning and teaching*. Oxford University Press.

Petrusa, E., Camp, M., Haward, D., *et al.* (1995). Measuring doctor—patient relationship and communication in a clinical performance examination. In *Proceedings of the Sixth Ottawa Conference on Medical Education*, (ed. A. Rothman and R. Cohen). University of Toronto Bookstore Custom Publishing, Toronto.

Poulton, J., Rylance, G.W., and Johnson, M.R.D. (1986). Medical teaching of the cultural aspects of ethnic minorities: does it exist? *Medical Education*, **20**, 492–7.

Rashid, A., Allen, J., Thaw, R. and Aram, G. (1994). Performance based assessment using simulated patients. *Education for General Practice*, **5**, 151–6.

Reid, A.L.A. (1993). The contribution of general practice to the medical curriculum. *Annals of Community-Oriented Education*, **6**, 115–23.

Rethans, J-J., Sturmans, F., Drop, R., *et al.* (1991). Does competence of general practitioners predict their performance? Comparison between examination setting and actual practice. *British Medical Journal*, **303**, 1377–80.

Ross, J.M. and Stanley, I.M. (1985). A system of affective learning behaviours for medical education. *Family Practice*, **2**, 213–18.

Royal College of General Practitioners (1970) A future in general practice. *Journal of the Royal College of General Practitioners*, **20**, Suppl. 1.

Royal College of General Practitioners (1972). *The future general practitioner*. British Medical Association, London.

Royal College of General Practitioners (1993). *Portfolio-based learning in general practice*. Occasional Paper 63. Royal College of General Practitioners, Exeter.

Schnabl, G., Hassard, T., and Kopelow, M. (1991). The assessment of interpersonal skills using standardised patients. *Academic Medicine*, **66**, S34–S36.

Schön, D.A. (1987). *Educating the reflective practitioner*. Jossey-Bass, San Francisco.

Schmidt, H.G. (1993). Foundations of problem-based learning: some explanatory notes. *Medical Education*, **27**, 422–32.

Seabrook, M., Booton, P., and Evans, T. (1994). *Widening the horizons of medical education*. King's Fund, London.

Seedhouse, D. (1988). *Ethics: the heart of health care*. Wiley, Chichester.

Simpson, M., Buckman, R., Stewart, M., *et al.* (1991) Doctor—patient communication: the Toronto consensus statement. *British Medical Journal*, **303**, 1385–7.

Skrabanek, P. and McCormick, J. (1992). *Follies and fallacies in medicine*. Tarragon, Chippenham.

Spence, J. (1960). *The purpose and practice of medicine*. Oxford University Press.

Stanley, I. M. and Al-Shehri, A. (1992). What do medical students seek to learn from general practice? A study of personal learning objectives. *British Journal of General Practice*, **42**, 512–16.

Stillman, P., Swanson, D., Smee, S., *et al.* (1986). Assessing clinical skills of residents with standardized patients. *Annals of Internal Medicine*, **105**, 762–71.

Stillman, P., Regan, M., and Philbin, M. (1991). Results of a survey on the use of standardized patients to teach and evaluate clinical skills. *Academic Medicine*, **66**, 271–2.

Stott, N.C.H. and Davis, R.H. (1979) The exceptional potential in each primary care consultation. *Journal of the Royal College of General Practitioners*, **29**, 201–5.

Sydenham, T. *The works*, Vol I. Quoted in Wartman W.B. (1961). *Medical teaching in Western civilization*. Year Book Medical, Chicago.

Tate, P. (1994). *The doctor's communication handbook*. Radcliffe Medical Press, Oxford.

Towle, A. (ed.) (1992). *Community-based teaching, sharing ideas 1*. King's Fund, London.

Tuckett, D., Boulton, M., Olson, C., and Williams, A. (1985). *Meetings between experts*. Tavistock, London.

Tutton, P.J.M. (1993). Medical school entrants—semistructured interview ratings, prior scholastic achievement and personality profiles. *Medical Education*, 27, 328–36.

Usherwood, T., Josebury, H., and Hannay, D. (1991). Student-directed problem-based learning in general practice and public health medicine. *Medical Education*, 25, 421–9.

van der Vleuten, C. and Swanson D. (1990). Assessment of clinical skills with standardised patients: state of the art. *Teaching and Learning in Medicine*, 2, 58–76.

van der Vleuten, C., Norman, G.R., and Graaff, E. (1991). Pitfalls in the pursuit of objectivity: issues of reliability. *Medical Education*, 25, 110–18.

Vu, N.V., Barrows, H., March, M., *et al.* (1992). Six years of comprehensive, clinical, performance-based assessment using standardized patients at the Southern Illinois University School of Medicine. *Academic Medicine*, 67, 42–50.

Walton, H.J. and Matthews, M.B. (1989). Essentials of problem-based learning. *Medical Education,* 23, 542–58.

Wharton, M. (1995). Clinical training in the community: a holistic approach. *British Medical Journal*, 310, 407.

Windeyer, B. (1966). University education in the twentieth century. In *The evolution of medical education in Britain*, (ed. F.J.L.Poynter). Pitman, London.

Wood, R. (1991). *Assessment and testing*. Cambridge University Press. Walton, H.J. (ed). (1993). *Proceedings of the World Summit on Medical Education, Medical Education*, 28 (Suppl. 1).

World Health Organization (1987). *Community-based education of health personnel*—Report of a WHO study group. WHO Technical Report, Series 746.

World Medical Association (1954). Proceedings of the First World Conference on Medical Education. Geoffrey Cumberlege, Oxford University Press, London.

Wykurz, G. (1992). The community module and beyond. In *Community-based Teaching, sharing ideas, 1, (ed. A.Towle). King's Fund, London.*

Index